The Galveston Diet Cookbook for Beginners

Nutritious & Mouthwatering Recipes to Alleviate Hormonal Symptoms and Combat Menopause, Starting Your Day with Breakfast Bliss.

Alonzo S. Wicks

Table Of Content

Introduction

Here in The Galveston Diet Cookbook for Beginners and we will change the way you eat for the better with a delicious adventure. Here and you will find more than just recipes; you will also get inspiration to lead a better life.

Picture yourself eagerly embracin' each new day and knowin' that this cookbook has the secrets to revivin' your health an' well being. This cookbook is for everyone and from seasoned chefs to those who are just gettin' their feet wet in the kitchen. Its goal is to help its readers make healthy and appetizin' meals that they will love.

This cookbook and however and is a testimony to the fact that food has the ability to cure an' feed not just the body but also the spirit. It's all about nourishin' ourselves with abundant natural resources an' usin' them to power ourselves.

Indulge your taste sensations while readin' up about the Galveston Diet and a science based lifestyle program that aims to improve your health an' wellness. From colorful salads that are burstin' with freshness to fillin' main dishes that will fulfill your appetite an' your spirit and every recipe is carefully planned to help you accomplish your health objectives without compromisin' on taste or pleasure.

This cookbook is full of delicious recipes and but it is also a love letter to friendship an' family. It's all about gatherin' with loved ones around the dinner table to enjoy good food and good company and an' tales. In the midst of the highs an' lows of our health journey and it is about creatin' a community where everyone feels welcome an' supported.

If you are travelin' with loved ones or by yourself and please, know that you are not experiencin' this journey alone. A community of individuals who are committed to helpin' you live your best life an' who will always have your back is what you'll find here and in addition to recipes.

Without further ado, let us delve into the gastronomic pleasures that lie ahead an' set out on a path to greater health and one tasty meal at a time. "The Galveston Diet Cookbook for Beginners" is your ticket to a world where health is more than just a passin' fad an' delicious food is the norm.

Understanding the Galveston Diet:

Gaining an appreciation for the Galveston Diet necessitates exploring a more comprehensive view of health than just focusing on weight reduction. The emphasis is on taking part in a way of life that prioritizes caring for one's physical, mental, and spiritual health. Consumption of nutrient-dense, complete foods with minimal processed and inflammatory components is central to the Galveston Diet. However, the food you consume is just part of the equation; your eating technique and frame of mind are as important.

In an effort to alleviate the metabolic shifts and hormonal abnormalities that often follow menopause and perimenopause, the Galveston Diet caters specifically to women's requirements throughout these life transitions. Dietary changes that promote hormonal balance and decreased inflammation may help with weight management and other symptoms including lethargy, mood swings, and brain fog.

A lifestyle concept that promotes self-care and empowerment, the Galveston Diet goes beyond just a mere food plan. By teaching people to pay attention to their bodies and enjoy every meal, it encourages them to eat more mindfully. Optimal health is the result of a combination of elements, including regular physical exercise, stress management, and sufficient sleep.

Since there is no "magic bullet" when it comes to healthy eating, the Galveston Diet places an emphasis on adaptability and longevity. People are encouraged to try several things and personalize them until they discover what suits their body and lifestyle the best. The Galveston Diet promotes self-determination in health by holding participants accountable for their own actions, whether that's via grocery shopping, cooking, or practicing mindful eating.

To fully understand the Galveston Diet, one must have a holistic perspective on health that prioritizes proper nutrition, balance, and self-care. Being proactive in our pursuit of a better, happier life involves acknowledging the significant influence that our diet, thinking, and lifestyle choices have on our overall health.

What is the Galveston Diet?

More than just a set of dietary rules, the Galveston Diet promotes a way of life that is based on ecological consciousness and preventative medicine. This nutrition plan focuses on hormonal balance and is based on the ideas put out by Dr. Mary Claire Haver, a board-certified OB-GYN who is deeply committed to enabling women to choose their own health outcomes.

In its most basic form, the Galveston Diet takes into account the specific hormonal changes that women undergo throughout the course of their lives and places an emphasis on providing the body with meals that are full of nutrients. It acknowledges that lifestyle variables such as stress, age, and hormonal changes may affect metabolism and general health and aims to tackle these issues by recommending dietary adjustments.

The Galveston Diet favors a moderate strategy that encourages long-term sustainability and general health, as opposed to many trendy diets that offer severe limitations or fast solutions. The program promotes a diet rich in fruits, vegetables, lean meats, and healthy fats while simultaneously stressing the need to control portion sizes and eat high-quality meals.

Particularly for women undergoing menopause or dealing with other hormonal imbalances, the Galveston Diet places a focus on promoting hormonal balance as one of its important principles. Dietary changes like adding omega-3 fatty acids and phytoestrogens may help balance hormones, which in turn can reduce symptoms like exhaustion, mood swings, and abnormal weight gain.

Aside from nutrition, the Galveston Diet advocates for other parts of well-being, such as exercise, sufficient sleep, stress management, and mindful eating. It promotes a more all-encompassing view of health by showing how crucial one's food, way of life, and general health are.

As a breath of new air in the health and nutrition industry, the Galveston Diet places an emphasis on education, empowerment, and self-care. It offers a road map to improving energy, mood, and vitality in addition to losing weight by recognizing and respecting the specific demands of women's bodies.

How Does the Galveston Diet Work?

Based on the idea of hormonal balance, the Galveston Diet—created by Dr. Mary Claire Haver—targets the changes that happen to women's bodies as they become older. By treating the root cause of hormone imbalances—which may impede weight loss and general health—the Galveston Diet takes a more comprehensive approach than many conventional diets that center only on calorie tracking or limited eating habits.

Crucial hormones that regulate metabolism, energy levels, and fat storage—insulin, cortisol, and estrogen—are the primary targets of the Galveston Diet's efforts to maintain these levels. The goal of the Galveston Diet is to enhance health and achieve long-term weight reduction by regulating hormones via food adjustments, intermittent fasting, and targeted exercise.

According to the Galveston Diet, consuming balanced meals is the best way to keep your hormones in check and ensure that your body gets all the nutrients it needs. Vegetables that are high in fiber and protein, lean proteins, and low-glycemic carbs are all part of this. Dieters following the Galveston Diet may improve their bodies' ability to use fuel and lessen inflammation—the latter of which is often associated with hormone imbalances and weight gain—by opting for nutrient-dense meals rather than processed ones.

One of the Galveston Diet's tenets is intermittent fasting, which aids in insulin regulation and fat loss. People may improve their insulin sensitivity, metabolic flexibility, and capacity to use stored fat for energy by include fasting intervals in their regimen. In addition to aiding weight reduction, this method may have other health advantages, such as less inflammation and better cognitive function.

The Galveston Diet stresses the need for frequent, individually tailored exercise in conjunction with food adjustments and intermittent fasting. Incorporating regular physical exercise, whether it's strength training or cardiovascular exercises, into your routine will help you achieve your weight loss and hormone-balancing objectives.

With an emphasis on women's specific hormonal requirements, the Galveston Diet provides a holistic strategy for optimal health and weight management. People may enhance their quality of life and reach their weight reduction objectives by fixing fundamental imbalances and making long-term adjustments to their lifestyles. The Galveston Diet encourages women to be proactive about their health by providing them with nutritious meals, a framework for intermittent fasting, and consistent exercise.

Benefits of the Galveston Diet:

By addressing one's health from every angle, the Galveston Diet promotes not only weight reduction but also general energy and longevity. It provides many significant advantages, including the following:

Stabilizing Blood Sugar Levels: The Galveston Diet may assist with this by promoting the consumption of low-glycemic foods and by advocating the strategic scheduling of meals. This may help people with diabetes or insulin resistance maintain more consistent blood sugar levels, which in turn improves energy and emotional stability by reducing the likelihood of dangerous spikes and crashes.

The Galveston Diet emphasizes long-term, sustainable lifestyle adjustments to promote weight reduction, as opposed to the short-term effects of fad diets. Achieving and maintaining a healthy weight is made easier by encouraging nutrient-dense diets and opposing excessively processed, sugary foods. This helps people avoid feeling hungry or deprived.

Decreased Inflammation: a number of long-term health issues are associated with chronic Inflammation, such as autoimmune diseases, heart disease, and arthritis. Eat plenty of anti-inflammatory foods like berries, leafy greens, and fatty fish, and cut less on pro-inflammatory items like processed meats and refined sweets, according to the Galveston Diet. The health of your joints, your heart, and your whole body may all benefit from reduced inflammation levels, which this can help bring about.

Improved Cognitive Function and Focus: The Galveston Diet improves focus and mental clarity by ensuring a continuous supply of nutrients to the brain and balancing blood sugar levels. There has been a significant decrease in mental weariness and brain fog among many diet adherents, along with improvements in mood, attention, and focus.

For better gut health, follow the Galveston Diet's recommendations for foods high in fiber, such as fruits, vegetables, and whole grains. Yogurt and fermented veggies are also great sources of probiotics. By doing so, you may support a balanced population of gut bacteria, which are essential for proper digestion, immune system function, and general wellbeing. Less likelihood of gastrointestinal problems, better absorption of nutrients, and better immunological function are all linked to a balanced gut flora.

An increase in energy levels is one of the many benefits of following the Galveston Diet, which consists mostly of complex carbs, healthy fats, and lean proteins. In contrast to diets that stress either calorie restriction or overtraining, the Galveston Diet emphasizes

providing the body with healthy, nutrient-dense meals to support peak performance and energy.

Cardiovascular Health: The Galveston Diet encourages heart-healthy eating patterns by highlighting omega-3 fatty acid-rich foods like walnuts, flaxseeds, and salmon and fiber-and antioxidant-rich foods like fruits, vegetables, and whole grains. Reducing cholesterol levels, blood pressure, and overall cardiovascular health all contribute to a lower risk of cardiovascular disease.

The Galveston Diet is an all-encompassing plan for health and wellbeing that promotes a healthy weight, increased energy, longer life expectancy, and a reduced risk of chronic diseases. Emphasizing the importance of eating nutrient-dense meals, controlling Inflammation, maintaining stable blood sugar levels, and encouraging healthy lifestyle practices enables people to own their health and live their best lives.

Chapter 1: Breakfast Recipes

Berry Blast Smoothie

Prep time: 5 minutes

Cook time: 0 minutes

Servings: 2

Ingredients:
- Mixed berries (strawberries, blueberries, raspberries)—1 cup of
- 1 ripe banana
- 1/2 cup of of Greek yogurt
- Half a cup of of almond milk (or milk of your preference)
- 1 tbsp honey (optional)
- Ice cubes (optional)

Instruction :
1. The first step is to put everything into a blender. Combine the berries, banana, Greek yoghurt, almond milk, and honey (if liked) into the mixture. Puree the mixture.
2. Mash until smooth and blended. After mixing one more to incorporate, add ice cubes if you want it cooler.
3. Once the smoothie is put into glasses, it should be served immediately. This nutrient-dense Berry Blast Smoothie is the perfect way to begin your day.

Avocado Breakfast Bowl

Prep time: 10 minutes
Cook time: 0 minutes
Servings: 1

Ingredients:
- ripe avocado
- 2.2 eggs
- Salt and pepper to taste
- Optional toppings: diced tomatoes, sliced bell peppers, chopped cilantro, crumbled feta cheese

Instructions:

1. Destine the avocado and slice it in half. In order to provide a bigger opening for the eggs, scoop off some avocado flesh from both halves.
2. Crack one egg into the pit of each avocado. Put salt and pepper on top, according to your preference.
3. Toast the avocado halves in a pan or other oven-safe dish.
4. Turn the oven on high heat (about 425 degrees Fahrenheit, or 220 degrees Celsius). When the eggs and avocado halves have been in the oven for 10–15 minutes, they should be cooked to your preference.
5. After cooking, take the avocado halves out of the oven and let them cool for a little.
6. Top each avocado half with your preferred toppings, such sliced bell peppers, chopped cilantro, diced tomatoes, or crumbled feta cheese, if you so want.
7. A healthy and tasty way to start the day is to serve the Avocado Breakfast Bowl right away.

Spinach and Feta Omelette

Prep time: 10 minutes

Cook time: 5 minutes

Servings: 2

Ingredients:

- 4 large eggs
- 1 cup of of fresh spinach, chopped
- 1/4 cup of of crumbled feta cheese
- Salt and pepper to taste
- 1 tbsp olive oil

Instructions:

1. To beat the eggs thoroughly, place them in a basin and whisk them together. Just add salt and pepper as you taste it.
2. Before heating the pan over medium heat, add the olive oil and stir to coat.
3. Wilt the chopped spinach by adding it to the pan and cooking for two or three minutes.
4. In a skillet, combine the spinach and the beaten eggs.
5. Keep the eggs in the pan for a minute or two or until they begin to set around the edges.
6. In order to allow the raw eggs to stream below, carefully lift the omelet's borders with a spatula and tilt the pan.
7. Evenly distribute the crumbled feta cheese over half of the omelette-half.
8. Toss the cheese gently with the remaining half of the omelet.
9. Add the cheese and continue cooking for another minute or two or until the eggs are done.
10. Before serving, slide the omelet onto a dish.

Banana Nut Overnight Oats

Prep time: 5 minutes

Cook time: 0 minutes

Servings: 2

Ingredients:
- 1 cup of of rolled oats
- 1 cup of of milk (dairy or plant-based)
- 1 ripe banana, mashed
- 2. A few tbsps of chopped nuts, such as almonds or walnuts
- 1 tbsp honey or maple syrup (optional)
- 1/2 tsp ground cinnamon
- Pinch of salt

Instructions:
1. To make the rolled oats, milk, mashed banana, chopped almonds, honey or maple syrup (if desired), ground cinnamon, and a sprinkle of salt, mix everything in a container.
2. Beat until fully blended.
3. After covering the bowl or jar, place it in the refrigerator for at least four hours, or overnight, for the oats to soak up the liquid.
4. Make sure the oats are mixed well in the morning, and add extra milk if needed for a thicker consistency.
5. After an overnight in the fridge, you may enjoy the oats cold or warm them up in the microwave or on the hob if you choose.
6. Nourish yourself with this tasty and healthy meal!

Veggie Breakfast Burrito

Prep time: 15 minutes
Cook time: 15 minutes

Servings: 4

Ingredients:

- 4 large whole wheat tortillas
- 8 large eggs
- 1 cup of of diced bell peppers (any color)
- 1 cup of of diced onions
- 1 cup of of diced tomatoes
- 1 cup of of chopped spinach
- 1 cup of of shredded cheddar cheese
- Salt and pepper to taste
- Olive oil for cooking

Instructions:

1. The olive oil should be heated in a big pan over medium heat.
2. Before they soften, which should take around 5 minutes, add chopped bell peppers and onions to the pan and sauté.
3. Before whisking in the salt and pepper, toss the eggs in a basin.
4. Put the sautéed vegetables and whisked eggs into the pan after taking it off the heat.
5. Cook the eggs until they are thoroughly cooked and scrambled, stirring occasionally.
6. Turn off the stovetop fryer when the eggs are done.
7. Get the tortillas warmed up in a different pan or the microwave.
8. In order to make the burritos, top each tortilla with some scrambled eggs.
9. Garnish the eggs with shredded cheddar cheese, chopped spinach, and sliced tomatoes.
10. Chill the tortillas and roll them up firmly to make burritos.
11. Take a bite while it's warm!

Coconut Chia Pudding

Prep time: 5 minutes
Cook time: 0 minutes
Servings: 2

Ingredients:

- 1/4 cup of of chia seeds
- 1 cup of of coconut milk
- 1 tbsp maple syrup or honey (optional)
- 1/2 tsp vanilla extract
- Fresh fruit or nuts for topping (optional

Instructions:

1. Blend together the chia seeds, coconut milk, vanilla essence, maple syrup, honey (if desired), and syrup.
2. Whisk the ingredients until they are well mixed.
3. Put the dish in the fridge to thicken the chia seeds by soaking up the liquid, which should take at least two hours (or better still, the whole night).
4. In order to prevent the mixture from clumping, stir it occasionally while it cools.
5. After the chia pudding has thickened to your preferred consistency, take it out of the fridge.

6. After giving it one more toss, spoon the custard onto individual serving dishes.
7. For garnish, feel free to use nuts, fresh fruit, or whatever else you want.
8. Try it cold for a refreshing taste!
9. For a healthy and satisfying start to your day, try these dishes!

Blueberry Almond Pancakes

Prep time: 10 minutes
Cook time: 15 minutes
Servings: 4

Ingredients:

- 1 cup of of all-purpose flour
- 2 tbsp granulated sugar
- 1 tsp baking powder
- 1/2 tsp baking soda
- 1/4 tsp salt
- 1 cup of of almond milk
- 1 tbsp lemon juice
- 1 egg
- 2 tbsp melted butter
- 1/2 tsp almond extract
- 1 cup of of fresh blueberries
- Cooking spray or additional butter for cooking

Instructions:

1. Get a large basin and whisk together the flour, sugar, baking powder, soda, and salt to make the dough.
2. Lemon juice and almond milk should be combined in a different basin. After 5 minutes, it will begin to curdle somewhat.
3. Incorporate the egg, melted butter, and almond essence into the almond milk mixture by whisking until all incorporated.
4. Simply blend the dry components with the wet ones by pouring the liquids into the dry ones and stirring. Avoid overmixing; a few lumps are OK.
5. Combine the blueberries with a gentle stir.
6. Spray or cover lightly with butter or cooking spray in a large pan or griddle that is heated over medium heat.
7. Put about a quarter cup of of batter onto the pan for each pancake. Give it a couple of minutes in the pan until you see surface bubbles and the edges begin to harden.
8. Turn the pancakes over and continue cooking for another minute or two or until the second side is golden brown.

9. When you've used up half of the batter, coat the pan with more cooking spray or butter and repeat.
10. While still warm, top each pancake with maple syrup, more blueberries, and chopped almonds, if you want.

Greek Yogurt Parfait

Prep time: 5 minutes
Cook time: 0 minutes
Servings: 2

Ingredients:

- 1 cup of of Greek yogurt
- 1 tbsp honey
- 1/2 tsp vanilla extract
- 1/2 cup of of granola
- Half a cup of of fresh berries (a mix of strawberry, raspberry, and blueberries, for example)
- Additional toppings: sliced almonds, shredded coconut, and honey drizzle are all optional

Instructions:

1. Mix the Greek yogurt, honey, and vanilla essence together in a small bowl.
2. In two separate dishes or glasses, spoon a layer of the Greek yogurt mixture.
3. Pour some oats over the yogurt, then top it with some fresh berries.
4. Once the bowls or glasses are full, repeat the layering, finishing with a touch of granola.
5. Sliced almonds, shredded coconut, or a drizzle of honey are some extra toppings that may be added if desired.
6. The healthy and tasty Greek yogurt parfait is ready to be enjoyed right away.

Quinoa Breakfast Porridge

Prep time: 5 minutes
Cook time: 15 minutes
Servings: 2

Ingredients:

- 1/2 cup of of quinoa, rinsed
- 1 cup of of water
- 1 cup of of milk (dairy or plant-based)
- 1 tbsp honey or maple syrup
- 1/2 tsp vanilla extract
- Pinch of salt
- Fresh fruit, nuts, and seeds for topping (optional)

Instructions:

1. In a small pot, mix the quinoa with the water and a little salt. Bring to a boil while cooking over medium-high heat.
2. Cook the quinoa for 12–15 minutes, covered, after it boils, or until it is tender and the liquid has been absorbed.
3. Include the milk, maple syrup (or honey), and vanilla essence; stir to combine. Add another three to five minutes of cooking time, stirring periodically, or until cooked through.
4. Just take it off the stove and let it a few minutes to thicken.
5. Warm the quinoa porridge and garnish with freshly chopped fruit, nuts, and seeds. Have fun!

Smoked Salmon Bagel Stack

Prep time: 10 minutes
Cook time: 0 minutes
Servings: 1

Ingredients:

- 1 whole grain bagel, sliced and toasted
- 2-3 oz smoked salmon
- 2 tbsp cream cheese
- 1 tbsp capers, drained
- Red onion slices
- Fresh dill or chives, chopped Lemon wedges, for serving (optional)

Instructions:

1. Divide the toasted bagel in half and top with cream cheese.
2. Place half of the bagel on top of the smoked salmon.
3. Place capers on top of the smoked salmon after layering.
4. Finish it up with some red onion slices.
5. Add some fresh chives or minced dill as a garnish.
6. If you want, you may squeeze some lemon juice on top.
7. To create a sandwich, top with the remaining half of the bagel.
8. Indulge in the scrumptious smoked salmon bagel stack right now!
9. Savour these delicious breakfast choices!

Cinnamon Raisin French Toast

Prep time: 10 minutes
Cook time: 10 minutes
Servings: 4

Ingredients:

- 8 slices of bread (preferably whole wheat or multigrain)
- 4 eggs
- 1/2 cup of of milk
- 1 tsp vanilla extract
- 1 tsp ground cinnamon
- 1/4 cup of of raisins
- To grease the pan, use either butter or cooking spray.
- A garnish of fresh fruit, powdered sugar, or maple syrup is always welcome.

Instructions:

1. Eggs, milk, vanilla essence, and ground cinnamon should be well mixed in a small dish.
2. After adding the raisins, stir them in until they are uniformly distributed.
3. Apply frying spray or butter to a large pan or griddle and set it over medium heat to preheat.
4. Toss the bread slices in the egg mixture, ensuring that each one is coated equally.
5. Grill or sauté the bread pieces in a pan for two to three minutes each side, or until they become a golden brown and are cooked through.
6. Serve hot with maple syrup, powdered sugar, fresh fruit, or any toppings you choose after removing the French toast from the griddle.

Egg Muffin Cup of of

Prep time: 10 minutes
Cook time: 20 minutes
Servings: 6

Ingredients:

- 6 large eggs
- 1/4 cup of of milk
- Salt and pepper to taste
- onecup of of chopped veggies (e.g., spinach, bell peppers, tomatoes, onions, etc.)
- 1/2 cup of of shredded cheese (optional)
- Cooking spray or oil for greasing the muffin tin

Instructions:

1. After spraying or oiling a 6-cup of muffin pan, bring it to an oven temperature of 350°F (175°C)..
2. All of the ingredients—milk, eggs, salt, and pepper—must be well mixed in a big basin.
3. Add the chopped veggies and shredded cheese (if desired).
4. Fill up each muffin pan three quarters of the way to the top with the egg mixture. Scoop it out evenly.
5. Before placing in the preheated oven, bake the egg muffin cup ofs for about 15 to 20 minutes, or until they set and have a little brown bottom.
6. Once baked, take the muffins out of the oven and let them cool for a few minutes before removing them from the pan.
7. The egg muffin cup ofs are delicious, warm on their own, or topped with salsa or spicy sauce for salsa lovers.
8. Delight in your mouthwatering breakfast preparations!

Apple Cinnamon Baked Oatmeal

Prep time: 10 minutes
Cook time: 35 minutes
Servings: 6

Ingredients:

- 2 cup ofs of rolled oats
- 1 tsp baking powder
- 1/2 tsp salt
- 1 tsp ground cinnamon
- 2 cup ofs of unsweetened applesauce
- 1 cup of of milk (dairy or non-dairy)
- 1/4 cup of of maple syrup
- 2 tbsp melted butter or coconut oil
- 1 tsp vanilla extract
- 1 apple, diced
- Optional toppings: chopped nuts, additional cinnamon, maple syrup

Instructions:

1. First, get your oven up to 375 degrees Fahrenheit (190 degrees Celsius). Mix the butter or nonstick spray and roll it out into a baking dish.
2. Second, beat the rolled oats, baking soda, salt, and cinnamon powder in a large basin.
3. Third, in a separate dish, mix the applesauce, milk, maple syrup, melted coconut oil or butter, and vanilla extract using a whisk.
4. Blend the wet and dry components by pouring the liquid into the dry and stirring until smooth.
5. Carefully incorporate the apple dice until evenly distributed throughout the mixture.
6. 6 Evenly distribute the muesli mixture into the baking dish that has been prepared.
7. After the oven is ready, bake the muesli for 35 to 40 minutes, or until the top becomes golden and it's set.

8. Take it out of the oven and let it cool for a little before cutting it into serving.
9. Garnish with chopped nuts, cinnamon, and maple syrup, if desired, and serve cold. Get some healthy and comforting apple cinnamon baked muesli and eat it!

Southwest Breakfast Wrap

Prep time: 10 minutes
Cook time: 10 minutes
Servings: 2

Ingredients:

- There are four eggs of medium size.
- 4/5 cup of of chopped bell peppers, any color
- One-fourth cup of of chopped onion
- 1/4 cup of of cooked black beans
- 1/4 cup of of shredded cheddar cheese
- 2 large whole wheat tortillas
- Salt and pepper to taste
- Optional toppings: salsa, avocado slices, sour cream

Instructions:

1. Use a whisk to thoroughly beat the eggs in a bowl. Season with salt and pepper to taste.
2. In a medium-sized nonstick skillet, heat the oil. Sweat for a couple of minutes, or until the onions and chopped bell peppers start to soften, in the skillet.
3. Toss in the beaten eggs with the peppers and onions in the skillet. While stirring periodically, cook the eggs until they are scrambled and fully cooked.
4. Pliable tortillas may be warmed for about 30 seconds in a separate pan or microwave.
5. Put the two tortillas in the middle and divide the scrambled eggs equally between them.
6. Add cooked black beans and shredded cheddar cheese on top of each serving.
7. Make wraps by folding the tortillas' edges over the contents and rolling them securely.
8. Garnish with sour cream, avocado slices, salsa, and serve right away.

Protein-Packed Breakfast Sandwich

Prep time: 5 minutes
Cook time: 10 minutes
Servings: 2

Ingredients:

- 4 slices whole grain bread
- 4 large eggs
- 2 slices cooked turkey bacon
- 1/2 cup of of baby spinach leaves

- 1/4 cup of of sliced tomatoes
- 1/4 cup of of shredded mozzarella cheese
- Salt and pepper to taste
- Cooking spray or butter for cooking

Instructions:

1. To begin, coat a pan lightly with cooking spray or spray it completely and place it over medium heat.
2. Once you're ready for fried, scrambled, or poached eggs, crack them into the pan and cook them according to your preference. Sprinkle with salt and pepper to taste.
3. Toast the pieces of whole grain bread until they get golden brown while the eggs are cooking.
4. Assemble the sandwiches when the eggs have cooked: Toast the bread and top each piece with cooked turkey bacon.
5. Place a cooked egg on top of each piece of turkey bacon. Cover with baby spinach leaves and sliced tomatoes.
6. Top each sandwich with shredded mozzarella cheese.
7. Create sandwiches by adding the remaining toasted bread pieces on top.
8. Quickly serve, and if desired, top with ketchup or spicy sauce for more flavor.
9. Indulge in your tasty and healthy breakfast selections.

Green Smoothie Bowl

Prep time:10 minutes
Cook time: 0 minutes
Servings: 2

Ingredients:

- 2 ripe bananas, frozen
- 1 cup of of spinach leaves
- 1/2 cup of of frozen pineapple chunks
- 1/2 cup of of frozen mango chunks
- 1/2 cup of of almond milk
- 2 tbsp chia seeds
- Toppings (optional): sliced strawberries, blueberries, granola, shredded coconut, sliced almonds

Instructions:

1. Blend together the frozen bananas, spinach, mango, pineapple, almond milk, and chia seeds. Stir in the mango and frozen bananas. Whisk until combined.
2. Step 2: Blend until the mixture is silky smooth; if necessary, add more almond milk.
3. Bowls should be filled with the green smoothie.
4. Four, garnish with sliced strawberries, blueberries, granola, shredded coconut, almonds, or whatever else you choose.
5. Have some right now and savor it!

Sweet Potato Hash Browns

Prep time: 15 minutes
cook time: 20 minutes
Servings: 4

Ingredients:

- 2 medium sweet potatoes, peeled and grated
- 1 small onion, finely chopped
- 2 cloves garlic, minced
- 2 tbsp olive oil
- 1 tsp paprika
- 1/2 tsp salt
- 1/4 tsp black pepper
- Optional: chopped fresh parsley for garnish

Instructions:

1. Before you begin, take a clean kitchen towel and wring out all the extra liquid from the shredded sweet potatoes.
2. 2.In a large bowl, dissolve the sweet potato grate with the chopped onion, garlic powder, paprika, salt, and black pepper and whisk to combine.Thoroughly combine.
3. Third, cook the olive oil in a big pan over medium heat.
4. Spoonfuls of the sweet potato mixture, pressed down lightly to form patties, should be added to the heated oil in the pan.
5. After about four to five minutes of cooking, turn the hash browns over and keep cooking until they become crispy and golden brown in color.
6. Severely drain the hash browns on paper towels to soak up any extra grease after removing them from the pan.
7. Add chopped fresh parsley as a garnish, if preferred.
8. With your preferred breakfast items, serve the heated sweet potato hash browns as dish number eight.

Mediterranean Scramble

Prep time: 10 minutes
Cook time: 10 minutes
Servings: 2

Ingredients:

- 4 large eggs
- one-fourth cup of of red bell pepper, diced
- one-fourth cup of of green bell pepper, diced
- 1/4 cup of of diced red onion
- 1/4 cup of of chopped spinach
- 1/4 cup of of crumbled feta cheese
- 2 tbsp chopped fresh parsley
- Salt and pepper to taste
- 1 tbsp olive oil

Instructions:

1. A bowl and a whisk are all you need to thoroughly beat the eggs. Sprinkle with salt and pepper to taste.
2. Melt the olive oil in a pan that won't stick under medium heat.
3. The next step is to put chopped red onion and bell peppers in the pan. Gently sauté until tender, which should take around three to four minutes.
4. Toss in the chopped spinach and sauté for a minute or two or until the spinach wilts.
5. Scatter the beaten eggs over the veggies in the pan.
6. Scramble the eggs gently with a spatula, stirring every so often, until they reach the consistency you want. 6.
7. Just before the eggs are about to be done, cover them with crumbled feta cheese and heat for another minute or until the cheese begins to melt.
8. Scatter chopped fresh parsley over the scramble and remove from heat.
9. Take a bite while it's hot!

Mango Coconut Yogurt Bowl

Prep time: 5 minutes
Cook time: 0 minutes
Servings: 1

Ingredients:
- 1/2 cup of of plain Greek yogurt
- 1/2 ripe mango, diced
- 2 tbsp shredded coconut
- 1 tbsp honey or maple syrup (optional)
- An additional tbsp of chopped nuts, such as walnuts or almonds, is always welcome.
- Fresh mint leaves for garnish (optional)

Instructions:
1. Begin by combining the plain Greek yogurt with a bowl.
2. Sprinkle chopped mango and shredded coconut on top of the yogurt.
1. Third, for a sweeter taste, you may drizzle maple syrup or honey on top.
3. If you'd like some added protein and crunch, you may sprinkle chopped nuts over the yoghurt dish.
2. Fifth, for a vibrant and revitalizing garnish, top with mint leaves.
6. Take a bite out of your cool Mango Coconut Yoghurt Bowl right now!

Almond Butter Toast with Berries

Prep time: 5 minutes
Cook time: 0 minutes
Servings: 1

Ingredients:

- 2 slices of whole grain bread
- 2 tbsps of almond butter
- Half a cup of of a variety of berries, including strawberries, blueberries, and raspberries
- 1 tbsp honey or maple syrup (optional)
- Pinch of cinnamon

Instructions:

1. Toast the whole grain bread pieces until they are as crunchy as you want.
7. Divide the almond butter among the bread and spread it evenly.
2. After washing, blot dry the mixed berries using a paper towel.
8. Fourth, put the almond butter on a plate. Top with the mixed berries.
4. If you'd like it sweeter, drizzle with maple syrup or honey.
5. If you want to add more flavor, sprinkle a touch of cinnamon on top.
6. Top with berries and serve right away to savor the healthy almond butter toast!

CHAPTER 2: LUNCH RECIPES

Grilled Chicken Caesar Salad Wraps:

Prep time: 20 minutes
Cook time: 10 minutes
Servings: 4

Ingredients:

- 2 boneless, skinless chicken breasts
- Salt and pepper to taste
- 4 large flour tortillas
- 2 cup ofs of romaine lettuce, chopped
- 1 cup of of cherry tomatoes, halved
- 1/2 cup of of grated Parmesan cheese
- Caesar salad dressing (store-bought or homemade)

Instructions:

1. Get the grill ready by heating it up to medium-high.
2. Be sure to season both sides of the chicken breasts with salt and pepper.
3. After the chicken has been grilled for four to five minutes per side, or until it is no longer pink in the middle, remove it from the grill.
4. After removing the chicken from the grill and slicing it thinly, step four is to give it a few minutes to rest.
5. Position the tortillas on a level surface.

6. Sixth, fill the tortillas with chopped romaine lettuce, dividing it evenly and placing it in the middle of each.
7. Place sliced grilled chicken, cherry tomatoes, and grated Parmesan cheese on top of the lettuce.
8. Toss the filling ingredients with the Caesar salad dressing.
9. Roll up the tortillas securely after folding in the edges.
10. Whether you're serving them right away or want to make them portable, wrap them securely in foil.

Quinoa and Black Bean Stuffed Bell Peppers

Prep time: 15 minutes
Cook time: 30 minutes
Servings: 4

Ingredients:

- 4 large bell peppers, any color
- 1 cup of of quinoa, rinsed
- 1 can (15 0zs) black beans, drained and rinsed
- 1 cup of corn kernels, thawed or unthawed
- one cup of of diced tomatoes
- 1/2 cup of of diced onion
- 2 cloves garlic, minced
- 1 tsp ground cumin
- 1 tsp chili powder
- Salt and pepper to taste
- A cup of of shredded cheese, preferably cheddar, Monterey Jack, or a combination of the two
- Fresh cilantro, chopped (optional, for garnish)

Instructions:

1. Start by getting your oven ready at 375°F or 190°C.
2. Step 2: De-seed and membrane the bell peppers after removing the tops.
3. In a large pan, heat some olive oil over medium heat.
4. Cook the minced garlic and chopped onion for two to three minutes or until they are softened.
5. Combine the corn, quinoa, black beans, chopped tomatoes, cayenne pepper, ground cumin, and salt. Stir periodically while it cooks for another 5 minutes.

6. Take the pan off the stove and melt half of the shredded cheese by stirring it in.
7. Put a little of the quinoa and black bean mixture into each bell pepper, pushing down gently with a spoon.
8. With the peppers upright, put the filled ones on a baking dish.
9. Turn the oven up to 375 degrees and bake for 25 minutes with the foil on.
10. After removing the foil, top the filled peppers with the remaining shredded cheese. Bake uncovered for 5 more minutes or until the cheese melts and bubbles.
11. Optional: For a garnish, you can top with chopped cilantro just before serving.

Indulge in these tasty and healthy meals!

Avocado Tuna Salad Lettuce Wraps

Prep time: 15 minutes
Cook time: 0 minutes
Servings: 4

Ingredients:

- 2 cans (5 oz each) tuna, drained
- 1 ripe avocado, mashed
- Finely minced red onion, 1/4 cup of
- quarter cup of of finely chopped celery
- 2 tbsps fresh lemon juice
- 1 tbsp fresh parsley, chopped
- Salt and pepper to taste
- 8 large lettuce leaves (such as butter lettuce or romaine)

Instructions:

1. Put the drained tuna, avocado, red onion, celery, lemon juice, and parsley in a big bowl and mix well.
2. Stir all the ingredients until they are thoroughly blended.
3. Season to taste with salt and pepper.
4. Spoon some of the avocado-tuna combinations onto a lettuce leaf for every lettuce leaf.
5. Wrap the lettuce leaves in a ball.
6. Quickly prepare and savor!

Mediterranean Chickpea Salad

Prep time: 10 minutes
Cook time: 0 minutes
Servings: 4

Ingredients:

- 2 cans of washed and drained chickpeas, 15 ozs of each.
- One cup of of cherry tomatoes, halved
- thinly sliced cucumber, one
- 1/4 cup of of red onion, roughly chopped.
- Half a quarter cup of of pitted Kalamata olives, also.
- 1/4 cup of of fresh parsley, chopped
- 2 tbsps extra virgin olive oil
- 1 tbsp red wine vinegar
- 1 0z dried oregano
- Salt and pepper to taste
- Feta cheese, crumbled (optional)

Instructions:

1. In a big bowl, combine the chickpeas, halves of Kalamata olives, cherry tomatoes, cucumber, red onion, chopped parsley, and the rest of the ingredients.
2. In another bowl, combine the red wine vinegar, dried oregano, salt, pepper, and extra virgin olive oil to make the dressing. Toss the chickpea mixture with the dressing until it is well covered.
3. Make any required adjustments to the seasoning by tasting.
4. After serving, top with crumbled feta cheese if you like.
5. Toss in the fridge and wait to serve or serve right away.
6. Nourish your body and taste buds with this revitalizing Chickpea Salad from the Mediterranean!
7. Have fun making these healthy and tasty dishes!

Turkey and Avocado Club Sandwiches

Prep time: 10 minutes
Cook time: 0 minutes
Servings: 2

Ingredients:

- 6 slices whole wheat bread
- 6 slices turkey breast
- 4 slices of cooked bacon
- 1 ripe avocado, sliced
- 4 lettuce leaves
- 2 slices tomato
- Mayonnaise (optional)
- Mustard (optional)
- Salt and pepper to taste

Instructions:

1. On a clean board, spread the bread slices.
2. If you'd like, you may coat half of the slices with a thin layer of mustard and mayonnaise.
3. Arrange the turkey breast, bacon, avocado slices, lettuce, and tomato on top of the pieces that have mayo and mustard.
4. Add pepper and salt to taste.
5. Place a slice of bread on top of each sandwich to finish.
6. Separate the sandwiches into three equal halves by carefully cutting them diagonally.
7. Enjoy right away after serving!

Veggie and Hummus Wrap

Prep time: 15 minutes
Cook time: 0 minutes
Servings: 2

Ingredients:

- 2 large whole wheat tortillas
- 1/2 cup of of hummus
- 1 cup of of mixed salad greens
- 1/2 cucumber, thinly sliced
- 1/2 bell pepper, thinly sliced
- 1/4 cup of of shredded carrots
- 1/4 cup of of sliced red cabbage
- Salt and pepper to taste

Instructions:

1. Begin by spreading out the tortillas on a spotless surface.
2. Second, top each tortilla with a thick coating of hummus.
3. In the middle of each tortilla, place the sliced red cabbage, mixed salad greens, cucumber, bell pepper, and shredded carrots.
4. Add pepper and salt to taste.
5. Gently fold the tortilla edges over the filling, and then secure the ends to create wraps.
6. Cut the wraps in half diagonally so you have two pieces.
7. You can either serve it right away or wrap it in foil to make it a portable dinner.
8. Take a bite out of your healthy and tasty Veggie and Hummus Wraps!

Shrimp and Vegetable Stir-Fry

Prep time: 15 minutes
Cook time: 10 minutes
Servings: 4

Ingredients:

- 1 lb large shrimp, peeled and deveined.
- chopped veggies (e.g., broccoli, snap peas, carrots, bell peppers) 2 cup ofs
- 3 cloves garlic, minced
- 2 tbsps soy sauce
- 1 tbsp sesame oil
- 1 tbsp olive oil
- 1 tsp ginger, grated
- Salt and pepper to taste
- Cooked rice or noodles for serving
- Arrange sliced green onions and sesame seeds on top, if d

Instructions:

1. Place olive oil in a big pan or wok and heat it over medium-high heat.
2. Then, to the same pan, add the grated ginger and minced garlic. Infuse with aroma and cook for 1 minute.
3. Add the shrimp to the heated skillet and cook for a couple of minutes or until they start to turn pink.
4. Add the mixed veggies and continue cooking for another 3 to 4 minutes, or until the vegetables are crisp-tender and the shrimp is opaque throughout.

5. 5-Mix the sesame oil and soy sauce in a small basin. After the shrimp and veggies are cooked, pour the sauce over them. Combine by tossing, and then heat for a further minute or two.
6. Season to taste with salt and pepper.
7. Seventh, top the stir-fried shrimp and vegetables with cooked rice or noodles.
8. Sesame seeds and sliced green onions can be used as a garnish if preferred.

Turkey and Quinoa Stuffed Peppers

Prep time: 20 minutes
Cook time: 40 minutes
Servings: 4

Ingredients:
- 4 large bell peppers, any color
- 1 cup of of quinoa, rinsed
- 1 ib lean ground turkey
- 1 small onion, diced
- 2 cloves garlic, minced
- 1 cup of of tomato sauce
- 1 tsp dried oregano
- 1 tsp dried basil
- Salt and pepper to taste
- 1 cup of of shredded mozzarella cheese
- Fresh parsley, chopped, for garnish (optional)

Instructions:
1. Let the oven heat up to 375°F, which is 190°C.
2. Scoop off the seeds and membranes from the bell peppers after removing the tops. After arranging the peppers in a baking dish, set them aside.
1. A medium saucepan should be heated to boiling point with 2 cup ofs of water. To make sure the quinoa absorbs all the water, simmer it covered over low heat for around 15 minutes.
3. Brown the ground turkey in a big pan over medium heat, making sure it's no longer pink. If necessary, remove any surplus fat.
4. In the same pan as the turkey, add the minced garlic and chopped onion. To soften the onion, cook it for two or three minutes.
2. After adding the cooked quinoa, tomato sauce, dried oregano, and dried basil, season with salt and pepper. Stir through. Just a couple more minutes in the pan should be enough to heat everything through.
8. Evenly distribute the turkey and quinoa mixture among the bell peppers that have been prepped.
9. Finish up the filled peppers by topping them with shredded mozzarella cheese.
10. Bake, covered with foil, for 30-35 minutes in a preheated oven or until peppers are tender and cheese is melted and bubbling.
11. Take it out of the oven and let it a few minutes to cool down before you dig in.
12. Add chopped fresh parsley as a garnish if you like.

Greek Yogurt Chicken Salad

Prep time: 15 minutes
Cook time: 20 minutes
Servings: 4

Ingredients:

- 2 boneless, skinless chicken breasts
- 1 cup of of Greek yogurt
- 1 tbsp lemon juice
- 1 tsp Dijon mustard
- 1/2 tsp garlic powder
- Salt and pepper to taste
- 1/4 cup of of diced cucumber
- 1/4 cup of of diced red onion
- 1/4 cup of of diced bell pepper
- 1/4 cup of of chopped fresh parsley
- 1/4 cup of of crumbled feta cheese
- Optional: pita bread or lettuce leaves for serving

Instructions:

1. Preheat an outside grill or a grill pan to medium-high heat.
1. Before you cook the chicken breasts, season them with salt and pepper.
2. Finally, grill the chicken for around 8 to 10 minutes per side to make sure it's cooked through and no longer pink in the center.
3. Prepare a bowl and combine the Greek yogurt, lemon juice, Dijon mustard, garlic powder, salt, and pepper. Stir until completely combined. After this, we reach the fourth step. Pour in and stir until well blended.
4. Remove from heat and let aside to rest for a few minutes. Slice into bite-sized pieces.
5. At last, add the feta cheese, diced bell pepper, chopped parsley, chopped chicken, sliced red onion, and diced Greek yoghurt. Coat all of the ingredients by tossing.
6. Serve the chicken salad alone or wrap it in lettuce leaves for a lighter alternative. Put it in pita bread if you like.
7. Chicken salad with Greek yogurt is tasty and nutritious.

Blackened Salmon Salad with Citrus Dressing

Prep time: 10 minutes
Cook time: 10 minutes
Servings: 2

Ingredients:

- 2 salmon fillets
- 1 tbsp olive oil
- 1 tbsp blackened seasoning (store-bought or homemade)
- Salt and pepper to taste
- 4 cup ofs of mixed salad greens
- 1/2 cup of of cherry tomatoes, halved
- 1/4 cup of of sliced red onion
- 1/4 cup of of sliced cucumber

- 1/4 cup of of sliced avocado
- One-fourth cup of of feta or goat cheese crumbles
- Citrus Dressing:
- 2 tbsps freshly squeezed orange juice
- 1 tbsp freshly squeezed lemon juice
- 1 tbsp olive oil
- 1 tsp honey
- Salt and pepper to taste

Instructions:

1. Gather your grill or pan and set it over high heat.
2. Second, make an olive oil coating and season the salmon fillets with salt, pepper, and blackened seasoning.
3. Grill the salmon for four to five minutes on each side or until it flakes easily when checked with a fork.
4. To prepare the citrus dressing, remove the orange and lemon juices from the dish and combine them with the olive oil, honey, salt, and pepper. Leave aside while you cook the fish. Get it off the heat.
5. Salad greens, avocado, cherry tomatoes, red onion, and cucumber should all be combined in a big salad dish.
6. Take the salmon from the grill and let it rest for a few minutes after frying. 6.
7. Seven, top each plate with half of the salad mixture and a cooked salmon fillet.
8. Add crumbled feta or goat cheese and a dab of citrus dressing on top of each salad.
9. Serve the Citrus Dressed Blackened Salmon Salad immediately and relish its vibrant colors and delicious flavors

Veggie and Lentil Soup

Prep time: 15 minutes
Cook time: 30 minutes
Servings: 4

Ingredients:

- 1 cup of of dried lentils, rinsed
- 4 cup ofs of vegetable broth
- 1 onion, diced
- 2 carrots, diced
- 2 celery stalks, diced
- 2 cloves garlic, minced
- 1 can (14 oz) diced tomatoes
- 1 tsp dried thyme
- 1 tsp dried oregano
- Salt and pepper to taste
- 2 cup of of spinach leaves
- 2 tbsps olive oil
- (Optional) Garnish with fresh parsley

Instructions:

1. First, in a large saucepan set over medium heat, melt the olive oil. Add chopped onion, celery, and carrots. To soften the vegetables, just sauté them for a few minutes.
2. To release some of the garlic's scent, sauté the minced garlic for another minute.
3. Next, mix the dried lentils, thyme, and oregano with the tomato juice.
4. When the water boils, add the vegetable broth. 4. The lentils will soften after 20 to 25 minutes of simmering covered over medium heat.
5. Season with salt and pepper to taste.
6. Just before serving, toss in the wilted spinach leaves.

7. Divide the soup among separate plates and garnish with optional chopped fresh parsley. Savor while the temperature is high!

Turkey and Spinach Quesadillas

Prep time: 10 minutes
Cook time: 10 minutes
Servings: 2

Ingredients:
- 4 large flour tortillas
- 1 cup of of cooked turkey breast, shredded
- 1 cup of of fresh spinach leaves
- 1 cup of of shredded cheddar cheese
- 1/2 cup of of salsa
- Cooking spray or olive oil for cooking

Instructions:
1. First, brush or spray an enormous pan with olive oil or cooking spray. Place the pan on a medium heat setting.
2. Press a tortilla flat and set it on the pan. Next, crumble some cheddar cheese over half of the tortilla.
3. On top of the cheese, you should place shredded turkey, fresh spinach leaves, and salsa.
4. Fold the tortilla in half lengthwise over the filling to form a half-moon.
5. Quesadillas should be cooked for a couple of minutes on each side, or until they are crispy and golden brown, while melting the cheese.
6. Step 6: Repeat with the remaining tortillas and contents.
7. Stop cooking the quesadillas when they're done and set them aside to cool for a minute. Slice them into wedges thereafter.
8. Serve hot, garnished with more salsa or fresh cheese. For dessert, try these quesadillas stuffed with turkey and spinach.

Roasted Vegetable and Quinoa Buddha Bowl

Prep time: 15 minutes
Cook time: 30 minutes
Servings: 4

Ingredients:
- 1 cup of of quinoa
- 2 cup ofs of water
- chopped veggies (e.g., zucchini, bell peppers, broccoli, and carrots)—2 cup ofs
- 2 tbsps olive oil
- 1 tsp garlic powder
- 1 tsp paprika
- Salt and pepper to taste
- 1 avocado, sliced

- 1/4 cup of of hummus
- Fresh cilantro for garnish
- Lemon wedges for serving

Instructions:

1. Gas mark 4, oven temperature 200 degrees Celsius.
2. Rinse the quinoa in cool water using a fine-mesh strainer.
3. Heat a medium pot of water until it boils. The quinoa should be cooked, and the water should be absorbed after washing it, so bring it to a simmer and cover it for about 15 minutes. After five minutes, remove from heat and cover to rest. Whisk to blend.
4. In the fourth step, arrange the chopped vegetables in a baking dish. Garlic powder, salt, pepper, paprika, and olive oil are the seasonings listed. Set aside until the quinoa is ready to be cooked.
5. In a preheated oven, roast the veggies for 20–25 minutes, tossing halfway through or until soft and slightly browned. Roast until done, then transfer to a preheated baking sheet.
6. For the Buddha bowls, divide the cooked quinoa into four separate dishes. Put roasted vegetables, avocado slices, and hummus in separate dishes and serve.
7. Top with chopped cilantro and add lemon wedges to each plate for a squeeze.

Asian-style Beef and Broccoli Stir-Fry

Prep time: 15 minutes
Cook time: 15 minutes
Servings: 4

Ingredients:

- 1 lb (450g) flank steak, thinly sliced against the grain
- 1/4 cup of of soy sauce
- 2 tbsps hoisin sauce
- 1 tbsp rice vinegar
- 1 tbsp sesame oil
- 1 tbsp cornstarch
- 2 tbsps vegetable oil
- 4 cup ofs of broccoli florets
- 2 cloves garlic, minced
- 1 tsp ginger, minced
- Cooked rice or noodles for serving
- Decorative sesame seeds and thinly sliced green onions

Instructions:

1. To begin, in a small bowl, mix together the cornstarch, beans, rice vinegar, soy sauce, hoisin sauce, and sesame oil. Turn off the heat.
2. 2 In a big skillet or wok set over medium-high heat, warm a tbsp of vegetable oil.
3. Third, brown the flank steak for two or three minutes in a single layer in the skillet after thinly slicing it. Once removed from the pan, set the steak aside.
4. Finish up the pan by adding the remaining tbsp of vegetable oil.

5. When the broccoli florets are somewhat softer and bright green, toss them into the pan. Reduce heat and simmer for three or four more minutes.
6. Keep the skillet and cook the broccoli and minced garlic for a minute or two more, turning often.
7. After the steak is done, return it to the pan and pour sauce over it. Platter alongside broccoli. Mix the sauce well to coat all of the ingredients.
8. Keep cooking for another two or three minutes after the steak is done, and the sauce has thickened.
9. The eighth stir-fry, which consists of spicy broccoli and beef, is best enjoyed with hot-cooked noodles or rice.
10. The dish is finished off beautifully with sliced green onions and sesame seeds. I wish you all the best!

Greek Couscous Salad with Feta and Olives

Prep time: 15 minutes
Cook time: 10 minutes
Servings: 4

Ingredients:

- 1 cup of couscous
- 1 ½ cup ofs water
- 1 cucumber, diced
- 1 cup of cherry tomatoes, halved
- ½ cup of Kalamata olives, pitted and sliced
- ½ cup of crumbled feta cheese
- ¼ cup of red onion, finely chopped
- ¼ cup of fresh parsley, chopped
- 2 tbsps extra virgin olive oil
- 2 tbsps lemon juice
- Salt and pepper to taste

Instructions:

1. 1 Boil water in a medium pot. Add the couscous, stir, then cover and take off the heat. After 5 minutes, fluff it with a fork.
2. Step 2: In a big basin, mix together the cooked couscous, cucumber, cherry tomatoes, olives, feta cheese, red onion, and parsley.
3. Third, mix the olive oil, lemon juice, salt, and pepper in a little bowl that is not part of the main bowl. Mix with a whisk.
4. Lightly toss the salad to coat all of the components with the dressing.

5. Enjoy right away, or let the flavors combine in the fridge for 30 minutes before serving. Have fun!

Chicken and Black Bean Burrito Bowl

Prep time: 20 minutes
Cook time: 25 minutes
Servings: 4

Ingredients:

- 1 cup of brown rice
- 2 cup ofs water or chicken broth
- 1 tbsp olive oil
- 1 ibslib boneless, skinless chicken breasts, diced
- 1 bell pepper, diced
- 1 small onion, diced
- Black beans, 15 oz. can (drained and washed)
- 1 cup of of corn kernels, either fresh, frozen, or from the can
- 1 teaspoon chilli powder
- 1 teaspoon cumin
- Salt and pepper to taste
- Optional toppings: diced avocado, shredded cheese, salsa, sour cream, cilantro

Instructions:

1. First, boil some water (or chicken broth) and brown rice in a medium pot. The rice should be soft, and the liquid should be absorbed after 15 to 20 minutes of simmering and covered over low heat.
2. Once the rice is done, transfer it to a large pan and, over medium heat, bring the olive oil to a simmer. After 6 to 8 minutes, chop the chicken breasts and put them back in the pan. Keep stirring the chicken every so often until it loses its pink color.
3. Saute the onion and bell pepper in the same pan as the chicken. After the first four to five minutes, continue cooking until the veggies are soft.
4. Combine corn kernels, black beans, chilli powder, cumin, salt, and pepper. Stir to combine. To heat thoroughly, cook for a further two to three minutes.
5. Spoon cooked rice into individual serving plates for the burrito bowls. Add the chicken and black bean mixture over top.
6. Top with salsa, sour cream, cilantro, sliced avocado, shredded cheese, and serve hot. Those healthy and tasty burrito bowls are yours to enjoy!

Caprese Salad with Balsamic Glaze

Prep time: 10 minutes
Cook time: 0 minutes
Servings: 4

Ingredients:

- 2 large ripe tomatoes, sliced
- 1 ibslib fresh mozzarella cheese, sliced
- 1/4 cup of fresh basil leaves
- Salt and black pepper, to taste
- Balsamic glaze for drizzling

Instructions:

1. First, on a serving tray, lay out the tomato and mozzarella slices in a pattern of alternating and slightly overlapping pieces.
2. Place a few leaves of fresh basil in the space between the mozzarella and tomato slices.
3. Third, include salt and black pepper in the salad as per your preference.
4. As a fourth step, dress the salad with the balsamic glaze.
5. Enjoy right away after serving!

Spicy Thai Peanut Noodles with Shrimp

Prep time: 15 minutes
Cook time: 10 minutes
Servings: 4

Ingredients:

- 8 ozs rice noodles
- 1 tbsp sesame oil
- 1 ibslib large shrimp, peeled and deveined
- 2 cloves garlic, minced
- 1 red bell pepper, thinly sliced
- 1 cup of shredded carrots
- 1/4 cup of chopped green onions
- 1/4 cup of chopped peanuts
- Lime wedges for serving
- Fresh cilantro leaves for garnish

For the sauce:

- 1/4 cup of creamy peanut butter
- 3 tbsps soy sauce
- 2 tbsps lime juice
- 2 tbsps honey
- 1 tbsp sriracha sauce
- 1 tbsp rice vinegar
- 1 teaspoon grated fresh ginger
- 2 cloves garlic, minced

Instructions:

1. Start by following the package directions for cooking the rice noodles. After draining, put it away.
2. 2 Make the sauce by whisking all the ingredients in a small bowl until they are smooth. Remove from the heat.
3. Heat the sesame oil in a big wok or pan over medium-high heat. Toss in the minced garlic and shrimp; cook, stirring occasionally, for two to three minutes on each side or until opaque and pink. Take the shrimp out of the pan and put them aside.
4. Shred some carrots and add some sliced bell pepper to the same skillet. Cook, stirring occasionally, for two or three minutes or until crisp-tender.
5. Combine the veggies in the pan with the cooked noodles and sauce. Coat everything evenly with the sauce and cook it thoroughly by tossing.
6. After the shrimp are done, put them back in the pan and mix them with the noodles and veggies.
7. Remove from the fire and top with chopped peanuts, fresh cilantro leaves, and chopped green onions.
8. Top with lime wedges and serve hot. Those shrimp and spicy peanut noodles from Thailand are delicious!

Mediterranean Veggie Pita Pockets

Prep time: 15 minutes
Cook time: 0 minutes
Servings: 4

Ingredients:
- 4 whole wheat pita pockets
- 1 cup of diced cucumber
- 1 cup of diced tomatoes
- 1 cup of sliced red bell pepper
- 1/2 cup of sliced red onion
- 1/2 cup of crumbled feta cheese
- 1/4 cup of chopped Kalamata olives
- 2 tbsps extra virgin olive oil
- 2 tbsps lemon juice
- 2 teaspoons dried oregano
- Salt and pepper to taste
- Fresh parsley for garnish (optional)

Instructions:
1. In a big basin, mix together pieces of diced cucumber, tomatoes, red bell pepper, red onion, crumbled feta cheese, and chopped Kalamata olives.
1. The dressing is made by mixing the dried oregano with salt, pepper, lemon juice, and extra virgin olive oil in a small dish. Incorporate by whisking.
2. Combine the vegetable mixture with the dressing and toss to coat.

3. For step four, soften the whole wheat pita pockets by warming them just a little.
4. Load the Mediterranean vegetable mixture into each pita pocket after carefully opening them.
5. Sprinkle some fresh parsley on top if you want.
6. Serve right away and enjoy these flavorful and revitalizing Veggie Pita Pockets from the Mediterranean!

Turkey and Avocado Spinach Wraps

Prep time: 10 minutes
Cook time: 0 minutes
Servings: 4

Ingredients:
- 4 large whole wheat or spinach tortillas
- 1 ibslib sliced turkey breast
- 1 large avocado, sliced
- 2 cup ofs fresh spinach leaves
- 1/2 cup of thinly sliced red onion
- 1/4 cup of plain Greek yogurt
- 2 tbsps Dijon mustard
- Salt and pepper to taste

Instructions:
1. On a spotless surface, spread out the tortillas made from whole wheat or spinach.
2) Evenly distribute one spoonful of Greek yogurt onto each tortilla.
3. Evenly distribute the tortillas with the sliced turkey breast, avocado, fresh spinach leaves, and thinly sliced red onion.
4. After filling each tortilla, drizzle with Dijon mustard.
Taste and add salt and pepper.
6. Carefully roll up each tortilla, being sure to fold in the edges.
7. Cut the wraps diagonally in half if you want, and then serve right away.
8. If you're looking for a healthy and portable lunch, try these Turkey and Avocado Spinach Wraps!

Chapter 3: Dinner Recipes

Lemon Herb Baked Salmon

Prep time: 10 minutes
Cook time: 20 minutes
Servings: 4

Ingredients:
- 4 salmon fillets
- 2 tbsps olive oil
- 2 cloves garlic, minced
- 1 lemon, zest and juice

- 1 tbsp fresh parsley, chopped
- 1 tbsp fresh dill, chopped
- Salt and pepper to taste

Instructions:

1. To make it ready to go, heat the oven to 375°F, which is 190°C. To get it ready to bake, grease or line a baking dish.
2. Spread out the baking dish and add the salmon fillets.
3. Stir the olive oil, garlic, lemon zest, lemon juice, parsley, dill, salt, and pepper in a small bowl.
4. Spread the mixture equally over the salmon fillets and pour it on top.
5. Poach the salmon for 20 minutes in a warm oven or until it flakes easily when tested with a fork.
6. When the salmon is done cooking, take it out of the oven and enjoy it hot. If you'd like, you may top it up with some extra lemon slices and fresh herbs.

Garlic Rosemary Grilled Chicken

Prep time: 15 minutes
Cook time: 15 minutes
Servings: 4

Ingredients:

- 4 boneless, skinless chicken breasts
- 3 cloves garlic, minced
- 2 tbsps fresh rosemary, chopped
- 1 tbsp olive oil
- Juice of 1 lemon
- Salt and pepper to taste

Instructions:

1. First, chop the rosemary and mince the garlic for the marinade. Put the lemon juice, olive oil, salt, and pepper into a little bowl.
2. Marinate the chicken breasts for two minutes in a shallow dish or a plastic bag that can be sealed. Coat the chicken well.
3. Marinating in the fridge for 30 minutes—or even 4 hours—will bring out the greatest taste.
4. Before setting aside, heat the grill to medium-high.
5. Set aside the marinated chicken breasts and remove them from the dish as the fourth step.
6. Grilling the chicken breasts for 5 to 6 minutes per side will ensure that they are cooked through and eliminate any pinkness in the center.
7. The sixth step is to take the chicken off the grill after it's cooked. Before slicing, let it a few minutes to rest.
8. Grill the chicken until it's hot and golden, then garnish with fresh rosemary sprigs, if desired.
9. Chew on some delicious stuff!

Shrimp Stir-Fry with Vegetables

Prep time: 15 minutes
Cook time: 10 minutes
Servings: 4

Ingredients:

- 1 ibslib shrimp, peeled and deveined
- 2 cup ofs of a variety of veggies (e.g., broccoli, snap peas, bell peppers)
- 2 cloves garlic, minced
- 2 tbsps soy sauce
- 1 tbsp sesame oil
- 1 tbsp olive oil
- 1 teaspoon grated ginger
- Salt and pepper to taste
- Cooked rice or noodles for servin

Instructions:

1. In a large wok or pan set over medium-high heat, warm the olive oil.
2. Saute the grated ginger and minced garlic in the pan for approximately one minute or until they release their aromatic aroma.
3. When the skillet is heated, toss in the prawns and cook for a couple of minutes or until they turn pink and opaque.
4. Toss in the blended veggies and continue to stir-fry for an additional three to four minutes or until they reach a tender-crisp texture.
5. Combine the sesame oil and soy sauce in a little bowl. Toss the prawns and veggies in the pan with the mixture.
6. Toss all the ingredients together to coat them evenly with sauce. If necessary, season with salt and pepper.
7. Top cooked rice or noodles with the prawn stir-fry and serve hot. Savour it!

Tex-Mex Quinoa Bowl

Prep time: 10 minutes
Cook time: 20 minutes
Servings: 4

Ingredients:

- 1 cup of quinoa, rinsed
- Veg broth or two cup ofs of water
- 15 oz of black beans, washed and drained from one can1 cup of of corn kernels (fresh, frozen, or canned)
- 1 avocado, diced
- 1 cup of cherry tomatoes, halved
- 1/4 cup of chopped fresh cilantro
- 1 lime, juiced
- 1 teaspoon ground cumin
- 1/2 teaspoon chili powder
- Salt and pepper to taste
- Optional toppings: shredded cheese, salsa, sour cream

Instructions:

1. Bring the quinoa and water (or broth) to a boil in a medium saucepan.

2. Turn the heat down to low, cover, and simmer for around fifteen to twenty minutes until the quinoa is cooked and the water has absorbed.
3. In a big basin, mix together the cooked quinoa, black beans, corn, avocado, chopped cilantro and split cherry tomatoes.
4. Lime juice, powdered cumin, chili powder, salt, and pepper should be whisked together in a small basin.
5. Stir the quinoa mixture with the dressing and stir until well incorporated.
6. If you think it needs more salt, pepper, or lime juice, adjust the seasoning to taste.
7. Spoon the Tex-Mex quinoa mixture into individual bowls and top with sour cream, salsa, shredded cheese, or anything you like.
8. Savour every bite of your Tex-Mex Quinoa Bowl, a healthy and delicious dish!

Mediterranean Stuffed Bell Peppers

Prep time: 20 minutes
Cook time: 40 minutes
Servings: 4

Ingredients:

- 4 large bell peppers (any color)
- 1 cup of quinoa, cooked
- One can of washed and drained chickpeas (15 ozs)
- 1 cup of cherry tomatoes, halved
- 1/2 cup of crumbled feta cheese
- 1/4 cup of chopped fresh parsley
- 2 cloves garlic, minced
- 1 teaspoon dried oregano
- Salt and pepper to taste
- Olive oil

Instructions:

1. Start by getting your oven ready at 375°F or 190°C.
2. After removing the seeds and membranes, slice the bell peppers in half lengthwise.
3. After the quinoa and chickpeas have cooked, combine them with the cherry tomatoes, feta cheese, parsley, garlic, and dried oregano in a big bowl. To taste, season with salt and pepper.
4. Insert the quinoa mixture into the peppers, being sure to push down slightly to compress the contents.
5. Arrange the filled bell peppers in a roasting pan. Pour olive oil over the top.
6. Place the dish in a warm oven and bake for 30 minutes, covered with foil.
7. After 10 more minutes of baking without the foil, the peppers should be soft, and the mixture should be hot.
8. Hot Mediterranean-filled bell peppers, topped with more parsley if desired, are served at number eight.

Spicy Thai Basil Tofu Stir-Fry:

Prep time: 15 minutes

Cook time: 15 minutes
Servings: 4

Ingredients:

- 14 ozs firm tofu, drained and cubed
- 2 tbsps soy sauce
- 1 tbsp sriracha sauce
- 1 tbsp sesame oil
- 2 tbsps vegetable oil
- 3 cloves garlic, minced
- 1 red bell pepper, thinly sliced
- 1 yellow bell pepper, thinly sliced
- 1 onion, thinly sliced
- 1 cup of fresh basil leaves
- Cooked rice for serving

Instructions:

1. Mix the cubed tofu with the sriracha sauce and soy sauce in a bowl. Allow it to soak for ten to fifteen minutes.
2. The second step is to heat the sesame oil and vegetable oil in a big wok or pan over medium-high heat.
3. Marinate the tofu for 5–7 minutes or until it becomes golden brown on both sides. Before setting aside, take the tofu out of the pan.
4. Transfer the minced garlic to the same pan and cook, stirring occasionally, for a minute.
5. Stir-fry the onion and bell pepper slices for three to four minutes or until they are soft and crisp.
6. Put the tofu back in the pan and top it over with the basil leaves. Toss in another two minutes of stirring to let the flavors blend.
7. Spoon the hot, spicy Thai basil tofu stir-fry over cooked rice and serve immediately.
8. Savor these tasty and appetizing dishes.

Cauliflower Fried Rice with Shrimp

Prep time: 15 minutes
Cook time: 15 minutes
Servings: 4

Ingredients:

- 1 head cauliflower, grated or finely chopped
- 1 tbsp sesame oil
- 1 onion, diced
- 2 cloves garlic, minced
- 1 cup of frozen peas and carrots, thawed
- 1/2 ibslib shrimp, peeled and deveined
- 3 tbsps soy sauce
- 2 eggs, beaten
- Salt and pepper to taste
- Green onions, chopped (for garnish)

Instructions:

1. First, in a large wok or pan set over medium heat, warm the sesame oil. Sauté the chopped onion and minced garlic until they release their delicious aroma.
2. Cook, stirring periodically, the grated cauliflower for 5 to 7 minutes, or until it begins to soften.
3. Move the cauliflower to the side of the pan and add the beaten eggs using the vacant space. Cook the eggs in a skillet until they're done, and add them to the cauliflower mixture.
4. Finally, toss in the shrimp with the frozen peas and carrots in the pan. Wait another three to five minutes, or until the shrimp become pink and are fully cooked.
5. Add the soy sauce to the cauliflower mixture and mix well. Make sure to season with salt and pepper according to your taste.
6. Serve after taking the skillet off the heat and topping with chopped green onions.

Balsamic Glazed Turkey Meatballs

Prep time: 15 minutes
Cook time: 20 minutes
Servings: 4

Ingredients:

- 1 ibslib ground turkey
- 1/2 cup of breadcrumbs
- 1/4 cup of grated Parmesan cheese
- 1 egg
- 2 cloves garlic, minced
- 1 teaspoon dried oregano
- 1/2 teaspoon salt
- 1/4 teaspoon black pepper
- 1/2 cup of balsamic vinegar
- 2 tbsps honey
- Chopped fresh parsley (for garnish)

Instructions:

1. Before you begin, get your oven ready for 400°F (200°C). Line a baking sheet with parchment paper.
2. Coat the ground turkey with the breadcrumbs, Parmesan cheese, egg, garlic powder, dried oregano, salt, and pepper in a big bowl. Whisk until well blended.
3. The next step is to shape the turkey mixture into meatballs that are approximately an inch in diameter. Once the baking pan is ready, set it aside.
4. To remove any pinkness from the center and get a golden brown crust, place the meatballs in a preheated oven and cook for fifteen to twenty minutes.
5. Make the balsamic glaze while the meatballs bake. Melt the honey and balsamic vinegar in a small pot. Keep tossing occasionally while you simmer for five to seven minutes over medium heat or until it thickens a little.
6. After the meatballs have cooked, take them out of the oven and pour the balsamic glaze over them.
7. Serve the meatballs with the glaze on top of a serving dish and garnish with chopped fresh parsley.
8. Cauliflower fried rice, shrimp, and balsamic-glazed turkey meatballs—a mouthwatering dish!

Creamy Coconut Curry Chickpeas

Prep time: 15 minutes
Cook time: 25 minutes
Servings: 4

Ingredients:

- 2 tbsps coconut oil
- 1 onion, diced
- 3 cloves garlic, minced
- 1 tbsp grated fresh ginger
- 2 tbsps curry powder
- 1 teaspoon ground turmeric
- 1 can (14 ozs) coconut milk
- 1 can (14 ozs) chickpeas, drained and rinsed
- 1 cup of diced tomatoes
- Salt and pepper to taste
- Fresh cilantro, chopped (for garnish)
- Cooked rice or naan bread (for serving

Instructions:

1. Place the coconut oil in a large saucepan and melt it over medium heat. 1. To soften, sauté the chopped onion for a further five minutes.
2. Season with the minced garlic and grated ginger, then simmer for 2 more minutes, stirring often.
3. In step three, toast the spices for an additional minute while mixing in the curry powder and powdered turmeric.
4. Pour the coconut milk into the mixture of onion and spices and stir to combine.
5. In a skillet, cook the chopped tomatoes and drained chickpeas together, stirring constantly.
6. Cook the curry at a low simmer for 15 minutes to let the flavors meld and the sauce thickens. Season with salt and pepper to taste.
7. Turn the curry off the heat when it reaches the thickness you want. 7.
8. Step 8: Spoon the coconut curry-flavored chickpeas over the naan or cooked rice. Sprinkle chopped cilantro on top.

Honey Mustard Glazed Pork Chops

Prep time: 10 minutes
Cook time: 20 minutes
Servings: 4

Ingredients:

- 4 boneless pork chops
- Salt and pepper to taste
- 2 tbsps olive oil
- 1/4 cup of honey
- 2 tbsps Dijon mustard
- 1 tbsp whole-grain mustard
- 2 cloves garlic, minced
- 1 tbsp apple cider vinegar
- Fresh parsley, chopped (for garnish)

Instructions:

1. To prepare the oven, bring the temperature up to 375°F, which is 190°C.

2. Season the pork chops with a generous quantity of salt and pepper on both sides.
3. Preheat the olive oil in a big oven-safe pan over medium-high heat. After the pan is hot, add the pork chops and brown them for two or three minutes on each side (turning once).
4. Mix the glaze ingredients (honey, Dijon mustard, whole grain mustard, chopped garlic, and apple cider vinegar) in a small bowl. Set aside while the pork chops are searing.
5. After the pork chops have been seared on both sides, be sure to cover each chop equally with the honey mustard glaze.
6. Preheat the oven to 145°F (63°C) and bake the pork chops in a pan for 12–15 minutes or until they are cooked through.
7. After taking the pan out of the oven, set aside a few minutes to allow the pork chops to rest before they are served.
8. Just before serving, top the pork chops coated in honey mustard with some freshly cut parsley. Savour it!

Ratatouille with Herbed Polenta

Prep time: 20 minutes
Cook time: 40 minutes
Servings: 4

Ingredients:

- 1 large eggplant, diced
- 2 zucchinis, diced
- 1 large bell pepper, diced
- 1 onion, diced
- 3 cloves garlic, minced
- 2 cup ofs diced tomatoes (canned or fresh)
- 2 tbsps tomato paste
- 2 tbsps olive oil
- Salt and pepper to taste
- Fresh basil leaves, chopped, for garnish

Herbed Polenta:

- 1 cup of polenta (cornmeal)
- 4 cup ofs water or vegetable broth
- 2 tbsps butter
- 1/4 cup of grated Parmesan cheese
- 1 tbsp fresh thyme leaves
- Salt and pepper to taste

Instructions:

1. A big pan should be heated over medium heat with the olive oil added to it. To soften, sauté the chopped onion for a further five minutes.
2. Cook for one more minute or until aromatic, then add the minced garlic.
3. Toss in the bell pepper, diced eggplant, and zucchini to the skillet. Ten minutes or so of cooking time, stirring periodically, should be plenty to tenderise the veggies.

4. Fourth, combine the tomato paste and diced tomatoes. Make your own seasoning blend using salt and pepper. Simmer the ratatouille for a further ten to fifteen minutes to let the flavors combine.

5. In the meanwhile, have the polenta herbed. Get the veggie broth or water boiling in a different saucepan. To avoid lumps, mix in the polenta slowly while stirring continuously.

6. Lower the heat to low and keep cooking the polenta, stirring often, until it thickens, which should take around 15-20 minutes.

7. Combine the eggs, milk, and thyme; then add the butter and Parmesan cheese. Make your own seasoning blend using salt and pepper.

8. Spoon the polenta with the herbs onto plates and then top with the ratatouille. Add some chopped fresh basil leaves as a garnish. Savour it!

Teriyaki Beef and Broccoli

Prep time: 15 minutes
Cook time: 15 minutes
Servings: 4

Ingredients:

- Thickly cut against the grain flank steak, weighing 1 ibslib
- 2 cup ofs broccoli florets
- 1 tbsp vegetable oil
- 3 cloves garlic, minced
- 1/4 cup of soy sauce
- 2 tbsps honey
- 1 tbsp rice vinegar
- 1 teaspoon sesame oil
- A mixture of 1 teaspoon of cornflour and 2 tbsps of water
- Decorative sesame seeds and thinly sliced green onions

Instructions:

1. In a modest bowl, whisk together the cornflour mixture, rice vinegar, soy sauce, honey, and sesame oil. Pop it out of the table.

2. Bring the vegetable oil to a boil in a large pan or wok. After about 30 seconds of cooking, or until the minced garlic begins to release its scent, toss it in.

3. Third, put a single layer of thinly sliced flank steak in the pan. After browning for one or two minutes without stirring, continue cooking for another two or three minutes while stirring occasionally. Take the meat out of the pan and put it aside.

4. Stir-fry the broccoli florets for two to three minutes, or until they are tender-crisp, in the same skillet.

5. Put the broccoli and cooked meat back into the pan. Coat the broccoli and meat equally with the teriyaki sauce.

6. After 1-2 minutes of cooking, the sauce should have thickened a little, and all the ingredients should be cooked thoroughly.

7. Once you're ready to serve, scoop the broccoli and teriyaki beef onto a platter. Onions and sesame seeds, cut, make a lovely garnish. Add heated rice or noodles on top while it's still hot. Savour it!

Lemon Garlic Butter Shrimp Pasta

Prep time: 15 minutes
Cook time: 15 minutes
Servings: 4

Ingredients:

- 8 ozs of pasta (linguine or spaghetti works well)
- Peeled and deveined big shrimp weighing 1 ibslib
- 4 cloves of garlic, minced
- 1 lemon, zest and juice
- 4 tbsps of unsalted butter
- Salt and black pepper to taste
- Fresh parsley, chopped, for garnish
- Grated Parmesan cheese for serving (optional)

Instructions:

1. Cook the pasta until it reaches a texture that is slightly firm, as directed on the package. Reserve half a cup of of the pasta in boiling water after draining.
2. While the pan is heated over medium heat, melt the butter. Once the garlic is aromatic, add the minced garlic and simmer for about 1 minute.
3. Third, sear the shrimp for two or three minutes on each side in a pan over medium heat or until opaque and pink.
4. Grind some black pepper, lemon zest, and salt into the shrimp.
5. Put the lemon juice into the pan and mix everything together. Give it a minute for the flavors to mingle.
6. Toss in the cooked pasta and a little of the pasta water you set aside into the skillet. Coat the pasta well with the lemon garlic butter sauce by tossing all of the ingredients together.
7. If necessary, adjust the seasoning according to your taste.
8. Add chopped parsley and grated Parmesan cheese as garnishes to the shrimp pasta and serve hot.

Mor can Spiced Lentil Soup

Prep time: 10 minutes
Cook time: 30 minutes
Servings: 6

Ingredients:

- 1 tbsp olive oil
- 1 onion, diced
- 3 cloves of garlic, minced
- 2 carrots, diced
- 2 celery stalks, diced
- 1 teaspoon ground cumin
- 1 teaspoon ground coriander
- 1/2 teaspoon ground cinnamon
- 1/2 teaspoon ground turmeric
- 1/4 teaspoon cayenne pepper (adjust to taste)

- Rinse and drain 1 cup of of dry red lentils.
- 4 cup ofs of chicken or veggie broth
- 1 (14-oz) can diced tomatoes
- Salt and black pepper to taste
- Fresh cilantro, chopped, for garnish
- Lemon wedges for serving

Instructions:

1. First, in a big saucepan, bring the olive oil to medium heat. About 5 minutes after adding the chopped onion, the onion should be softened.
2. Throw in the chopped carrots and celery, along with the minced garlic. Keep co king for another three to four minutes, or until the veggies become somewhat sof er.
3. Add the ground spices: cumin, coriander, cinnamon, turmeric, and cayenne pepper. Mix well. Infuse with aroma and cook for 1 minute.
4. Place the red lentils that have been washed into the saucepan along with the vegetable or chicken broth, hopped to atoms, and their juices. Combine by stirring
5. Simmer the soup, then cover and lower the heat to low. After twenty to twenty-five minutes, the lentils should be soft.
6. Add salt and black pepper to the soup according to your taste.
7. To add a Moroccan touch to the lamb soup, garnish it with chopped cilantro and sprinkle some fresh lemon juice. Heat and serve immediately.
8. Savor these tasty and appetizing meals!

Pesto Zucchini Noodles with Grilled Chicken

Prep time: 15 minutes
Cook time: 15 min tes
Servings: 4

Ingredients:

- 4 medium zucchinis, spiralized into noodles
- boneless, skinless chicken breasts
- Salt and pepper to taste
- 1 tbsp olive oil
- ½ cup of basil pesto
- ½ cup of cherry tomatoes, halved
- Grated Parmesan cheese for garnish
- Fresh basil leaves for garnish

Instructions:

1. Let the grill heat up to medium-high.
2. Put some pepper and salt on the chicken breasts.
3. 3–6 minutes on each side or until chicken is cooked through while grilli g. Lay it flat for a few minutes after taking it from the grill, and then slice it.
4. Melt the olive oil in a big pan over medium heat. After two or three minute of cooking, throw in the zucchini noodles and continue cooking until they are just soft.
5. Place cooked zucchini noodles in a big basin.
6. Add the grilled chicken, cherry tomatoes, and basil pesto to the zucchini noodles in a bowl.
7. Toss until the pesto is well distributed and all ingredients are covered.

8. Spoon the grilled chicken and pesto zucchini noodles onto individual dishes.
9. To with fresh basil leaves and grated Parmesan cheese.
10. Enjoy right away after serving!

Black Bean and Sweet Potato Enchiladas

Prep time: 20 minutes
Co k time: 30 minutes
Servings: 6

Ingredients:

- 2 medium sweet potatoes, peeled and diced
- 15 oz of black beans, washed and drained from one can
- one cup of of corn kernels (fresh, frozen, or canned)
- 1 teaspoon ground cumin
- 1 teaspoon chili powder
- Salt and pepper to taste
- 1 cup of enchilada sauce
- 12 small corn tortillas
- 1 cup of shredded cheese (cheddar, Monterey Jack, or a blend)
- fresh cilantro chopped for decoration
- Toppings: sour cream or Greek yogurt (not required)

Instructions:

1. Set oven temperature to 190°C, or 375°F. Butter a 9 x 13-inch baking pan.
2. Toss in the sweet potatoes and microwave for 3–4 minutes, or until just cooked, in a bowl that is safe to use in the microwave.
3. Combine cooked sweet potatoe , black beans, corn kernels, chilli powder, powdered cumin, salt and pepper in a sizable mixing dish. Mix thoroughly by stirring.
4. Spread a little quantity of enchilada sauce evenly over the bottom of the baking dish that you have prepared.
5. To make the corn tortillas more malleable, briefly reheat them in the microwave.
6. After spooning some of the black bean and sweet potato mixture onto each tortilla, fold it up and place it seam-side down in the baking dish.
7. Once the baking dish is full, keep stuffing and rolling the remaining tortillas.
8. Evenly distribute the leftover enchilada sauce on top of the enchiladas.
9. Top the enchiladas with some cheese that has been shredded.
10. Bake the baking dish in the preheated oven for 20 minutes while covering it with foil.
11. Take off the foil and bake for a further ten minutes or until the cheese is bubbling and melted.
12. Take it out of the oven and allow it to cool down for a s ort while before serving.
13. Top with freshly chopped cilantro and serve with Greek yogurt or sour cream, if preferred.
14. Savour your mouthwatering Enchiladas with Sweet Potato and Blac Beans!

Greek-Style Grilled Lamb Chops

Prep time: 15 minutes
Cook time: 10 minutes
Servings: 4

Ingredients:

- 8 lamb loin chops
- 1/4 cup of olive oil
- 3 cloves garlic, minced d
- 2 tbsps lemon juice
- 1 teaspoon dried oregano
- 1/2 teaspoon dried thyme
- Salt and pepper to taste
- Lemon wedges for serving
- Chopped fresh parsley for garnish

Instructions:

1. Combine the olive oil, lemon juice, minced garlic, dried thyme, dried oregano, salt, and pepper in a small bowl.
2. Put the lamb chops in a plastic bag that can be sealed or in a shallow plate. Make sure the chops are thoroughly coated by pouring the marinade over them.Refri erate the container for a minimum of one hour, ideally overnight, then cover and seal it for best results.
3. Set the grill's temperature to medium-high.
4. Take the lamb chops out of the marinade, throwing away any extra marinade.
5. Grill the lamb chops for 3 to 4 minutes on each side for medium-rare to attain the right doneness.
6. Before serving, take the lamb chops off the grill and giv them a few minutes to rest.
7. Garnish the grilled lamb chops with freshly cut parsley and serve with lemon wedges.

Tomato Basil Quinoa Risotto

Prep time: 10 minutes
Cook time: 25 minutes
Servings: 4

Ingredients:

- 1 cup of quinoa, rinsed
- 2 cup ofs vegetable broth
- 1 tbsp oli e oil
- 1 onion, finely chopped
- 2 cloves garlic, minced
- 1 cup of cherry tomatoes, halved
- 1/4 cup of chopped fresh basil
- Salt and pepper to taste
- Grated Parmesan cheese for serving (optional)

Instructions:

1. Place the vegetable broth in a medium saucepan and heat it to a simmer.
2. Heat the olive oil in a second, sizable skillet or saucepan over medium heat. Cook th chopped onion and garlic for around three minutes, or until they become s ft.
3. Place the washed quinoa in the skillet and toss often while toasting it for one to two minutes.
4. Stir the quinoa often and let it absorb the liquid before adding more as you gradually add the simmering vegetable broth, about 1/2 cup of at a time. Continue cooking for

another 20 minutes or more or until the quinoa is soft and the stock has been fully absorbed.

5. Add the chopped fresh basil and cherry tomatoes that have been halved. Simmer the tomatoes for a further two to three minutes, or until they begin to soften.
1. 6 Add salt and pepper to taste when preparing the quinoa risotto.
6. Pr sent the hot quinoa and tomato basil risotto, with the option to garnish it with grated P parmesan cheese.
2. Savor your flavorful tomato basil quinoa risotto with lamb chops cooked in Greek style!

Sesame Ginger Tofu Stir-Fry

Prep Time: 10 Minutes
Cook Time: 20 Minutes
Servings: 4

Ingredients:

- One diced 14-oz serving of extra-firm tofu
- 3 tbsps of cornstarch
- A quarter teaspoon of salt
- A spoonful of olive oil
- quarter cup of of broccoli florets, chopped
- the chopped florets of 1/4 cup of of broccoli
- A dish of 2 cup ofs of cooked brown rice
- Spicy Ginger Sesame Sauce
- three cloves of minced garlic
- 2 teaspoons of freshly grated ginger
- 3/4 teaspoon of maple syrup
- To make it gluten-free, you'll need 1/3 cup of of low-sodium soy sauce or tamari.
- 2 teaspoons of water
- two teaspoons of sesame oil that has been toasted
- Two teaspoons of rice vinegar

Instructions:

1. You have a few options for pressing the tofu: a tofu press, a kitchen towel or paper towels, and anything heavy. Give it a good 10 minutes to settle while you make the sauce and slice the veggies.
2. Toss the cubed tofu with the cornstarch and salt until it is well covered.
3. Before setting aside, whisk together the following sauce ingredients: garlic, ginger, maple syrup, soy sauce, water, sesame oil, and rice wine vinegar.
4. While the oil is heating in a big pan over medium heat, add the tofu. Allow to fry for two to three minutes or until crispy. After that, turn and cook for another two to three minutes or until golden brown throughout. Saute the tofu till it becomes caramelized, then add 2 tbsps of sauce.
5. After taking the tofu out of the pan, add a further teaspoon or two of olive oil. After waiting around five to seven minutes, add the carrots and broccoli and stir-fry until the veggies are soft. After the tofu is done, add the sauce and continue cooking for another minute or two or until the sauce has largely been absorbed.
6. Complement with cooked brown rice.

Butternut Squash and Kale Lasagna

Prep Time: 30 Mins
Cook Time: 45 Mins
Serves: 6-8

Ingredients:

Filling

- 1 medium butternut squash, cooked and cooled*
- 15 oz. ricotta cheese
- 3 cup ofs shredded mozzarella cheese
- 1 tsp. Salt
- ½ tsp. ground black pepper
- 1 tsp. garlic powder
- 1 tsp. onion powder
- ½ tsp. ground dried thyme
- 1 lb. Italian sausage (optional)
- 2 tbsp. olive oil
- 1 bunch kale, stems removed, chopped

Sauce

- 3 tbsp. butter
- 4 tbsp. flour
- 2 cup ofs vegetable broth
- 1 cup of milk
- ½ cup of heavy cream
- ½ cup of shredded parmesan cheese
- ½ tsp. salt
- ¼ tsp. ground black pepper
- No-boil lasagna noodles

Instructions:

1. The first step, after halving the butternut squash, is to collect a big bowl. You may season it with salt, pepper, garlic powder, onion powder, and thyme. First, mix the ricotta with the shredded mozzarella; set aside 1 cup of. Remove from the equation.
2. If used, brown the Italian sausage in a big skillet. Before you add it to the lasagna, heat the olive oil in a pan if you're following a vegetarian diet. Brown the sausage or heat the olive oil; next, sauté the greens until it wilts. Remove from the heat.
3. To melt the butter, a medium heat is ideal. Whisk the flour until well combined. To make a thick sauce, bring to a simmer over low heat and stir periodically. Toss in the vegetables, heavy cream, vegetable broth, and parmesan sauce. Finish with a pinch of pepper and salt.
4. An oven temperature of 350 degrees Fahrenheit must be preheated. A 13 by 9-inch baking dish should be coated with nonstick cooking spray. An even coating of sauce should cover the pan's base before you add three lasagna noodles. After you've layered the noodles with the butternut squash and cheese mixture, top with a little of the kale and sausage combination. Next, top with a couple of scoops of sauce and a tiny handful of the leftover mozzarella. Keep on until you've used all of the ingredients. The remaining sauce and mozzarella cheese should be layered on top of the last layer of lasagna noodles.
5. The lasagna may be chilled now until baking time.
6. In a preheated oven, bake until bubbling and brown, about 45 to 50 minutes.
7. Allow flavors to develop by setting aside for 30 minutes. Then, chop and serve.

Chapter 4: Snacks And Sides

Zesty Guacamole:

Prep Time: 10 minutes
Cook Time: 0 min
Servings: 4

Ingredients:

- 2 ripe avocados
- 1 small red onion, finely diced
- 1 medium tomato, diced
- 1 jalapeno pepper, seeded and minced
- 2 tbsps freshly squeezed lime juice
- 2 cloves garlic, minced
- 1/4 cup of fresh cilantro, chopped
- Salt and pepper to taste

Instructions:

1. Halve the avocados and scoop out their pits. Gather the meat and place it in a mixing basin.
2. Grind the avocados to a smooth consistency, leaving some texture intact, using a fork.
3. Toss the mashed avocados with the diced onion, tomato, jalapeño pepper, lime juice, minced garlic, and chopped cilantro.
4. Salt and pepper to taste.
5. Combine all of the ingredients by stirring them together.
6. If necessary, adjust the seasoning by tasting.
1. Tacos, salads, or sandwiches can be topped with this salsa, and it's best served soon with tortilla chips.

Crispy Baked Sweet Potato Fries:

Prep Time: 10 minutes
Cook Time: 25-30 minutes
Servings: 4

Ingredients:

- Peel and slice two big sweet potatoes into fries.
- 2 tbsps olive oil
- 1 teaspoon garlic powder
- 1 teaspoon paprika
- 1/2 teaspoon ground cumin
- Salt and pepper to taste

Instructions:

2. Position a baking sheet on top of the oven rack and heat it to 425°F, or 220°C.
3. Pour olive oil, garlic powder, paprika, cumin, salt, and pepper over the sweet potato fries in a big bowl. Toss to coat.
4. Preheat a baking sheet and spread the seasoned sweet potato fries evenly, leaving room between each fry.
5. Preheat oven to 25-30 minutes. Cook, stirring once, until the fries are crisp and golden.
6. Take it out of the oven and let it a few minutes to cool down before you dig in.
7. Enjoy when hot and top with your preferred dipping sauce.
8. Savor the flavorful guacamole and crunchy sweet potato fries.

Spinach and Artichoke Dip

Prep Time: 10 minutes
Cook Time: 25 minutes
Servings: 6

Ingredients:

- thawed and drained one 10-oz bag of frozen chopped spinach
- One 14-oz can of chopped and drained artichoke hearts
- 1 cup of of grated Parmesan cheese
- 1 cup of shredded mozzarella cheese
- 1/2 cup of mayonnaise
- 1/2 cup of sour cream
- 1 clove garlic, minced
- Salt and pepper to taste
- Tortilla chips or crackers for serving

Ingredients:

1. Bring the oven temperature up to 375°F, which is around 190°C.
2. Toss the chopped artichoke hearts, spinach, Parmesan, mozzarella, mayonnaise, sour cream, and minced garlic in a large basin. Stir until incorporated.
3. Third, add salt and pepper just before serving.
4. Level out a baking dish and pour in the batter.
5. After 20 to 25 minutes of preheating, the dip should be bubbling and have a golden brown top.
6. Serve after 6 minutes of cooling from the oven.
7. Garnish with tortilla chips or crackers and serve warm.

Caprese Skewers

Prep Time: 15 minutes
Cook Time: 0 minutes
Servings: 6

Ingredients:

- 1 pint cherry tomatoes
- 1 (8 oz) package fresh mozzarella cheese, cut into bite-sized pieces
- Fresh basil leaves
- Balsamic glaze (optional)
- Wooden skewers

Instructions:

1. First, give the basil leaves and cherry tomatoes a good wash.
2. Continue threading the items onto the skewers until all of the cherry tomatoes, mozzarella cheese, and basil leaves have been utilized.
3. Place a serving dish on top of the skewers.
4. just before serving, sprinkle with balsamic glaze if you want.
5. Enjoy as a quick snack or appetizer right away.

Buffalo Cauliflower Bites

Prep Time: 15 minutes
Cook Time: 25 minutes
Servings: 4

Ingredients:
- 1 head cauliflower, cut into florets
- 1/2 cup of all-purpose flour
- 1/2 cup of water
- 1 teaspoon garlic powder
- 1/2 teaspoon salt
- 1/4 teaspoon black pepper
- 1/2 cup of buffalo sauce
- 2 tbsps unsalted butter, melted

Instructions:
1. Turn the oven on high (450°F, 230°C). Put parchment paper on a baking pan.
2. In a big basin, blend the flour, water, garlic powder, salt, and black pepper until combined.
3. The next step is to coat the cauliflower florets uniformly with batter.
4. Spread out the cauliflower on the prepared baking sheet in a single layer.
5. Cook in the oven for 20 to 25 minutes or until crisp and golden.
6. Combine the melted butter and buffalo sauce in a small dish.
7. Take the cauliflower out of the oven and cover it well with the buffalo sauce mixture.
8. Top with your preferred dipping sauce and serve hot.

Mediterranean Hummus Platter

Prep Time: 10 minutes
Cook Time: 0 minutes
Servings: 4

Ingredients:
- 1 cup of hummus
- 1/2 cup of cherry tomatoes, halved
- 1/2 cup of cucumber, sliced
- 1/4 cup of Kalamata olives
- 1/4 cup of crumbled feta cheese
- 2 tbsps chopped fresh parsley
- 2 tbsps extra virgin olive oil
- Salt and black pepper to taste

- Pita bread or crackers for serving

Instructions:

1. On a serving dish, spread the hummus.
2. After the hummus has been mixed, top with cucumber slices, crumbled feta cheese, Kalamata olives, and cherry tomatoes.
3. Pour EVOO over the serving plate.
4. Add salt and black pepper according to your taste.
5. Top with some freshly chopped parsley.
1. Pita bread or crackers can be served as a side accompaniment

Parmesan Garlic Roasted Broccoli

Prep time: 10 minutes
Cook time: 20 minutes
Servings: 4

Ingredients:

- 1 head of broccoli, cut into florets
- 2 tbsps olive oil
- 2 cloves garlic, minced
- 1/4 cup of grated Parmesan cheese
- Salt and pepper to taste

Instructions:

2. Warming up the oven to 400°F (200°C) is the recommended temperature.
3. Toss the broccoli florets in a big basin with olive oil, pepper, garlic powder, Parmesan cheese, and salt until uniformly covered.
4. Distribute the coated broccoli equally on a baking sheet lined with paper.
5. To get crispy edges and soft broccoli, roast in a preheated oven for around fifteen to twenty minutes.
6. As a tasty accompaniment, serve hot.

Avocado Toast with Tomato and Basil

Prep time: 5 minutes
Cook time: 0 minutes
Servings: 2

Ingredients:

- 2 slices of whole grain bread, toasted
- 1 ripe avocado
- 1 small tomato, sliced
- 4-6 fresh basil leaves
- Salt and pepper to taste

Instructions:

1. Split the ripe avocado lengthwise and remove its meat onto a small dish. For a smooth avocado, use a fork to mash it.
2. Evenly distribute the mashed avocado over the pieces of toasted whole grain bread.
3. Sprinkle some fresh basil leaves and tomato slices on top of the avocado toast.
4. Season to taste with salt and pepper.
5. Serve immediately for a nutritious and tasty snack or breakfast.

Stuffed Mini Bell Peppers

Prep time: 20 minutes
Cook time: 20 minutes
Servings: 4

Ingredients:
- 12 mini bell peppers
- 1 cup of cooked quinoa
- 1 cup of black beans, drained and rinsed
- 1 cup of corn kernels (fresh or frozen)
- 1/2 cup of diced tomatoes
- 1/4 cup of diced red onion
- 1/4 cup of chopped fresh cilantro
- 1 teaspoon ground cumin
- 1 teaspoon chili powder
- Salt and pepper to taste
- 1 cup of shredded cheese (optional)
- Sliced green onions for garnish

Instructions:
1. Start by getting your oven ready at 375°F or 190°C. Arrange a baking sheet with parchment paper.
2. After halves of each little bell pepper, cut off the tops and discard the seeds and membranes.
3. In a large basin, mix together the quinoa, black beans, corn, diced tomatoes, red onion, cilantro, ground cumin, chili powder, salt, and pepper. Incorporate by rolling on evenly.
4. Gently push down on each small bell pepper to stuff it with the quinoa mixture.
5. Once the peppers are filled, top with cheese if desired.
6. After preparing the baking sheet, put the filled peppers on it. After 15–20 minutes of baking in a preheated oven, the peppers should be tender, and the filling should be fully cooked.
7. After cooking is complete, take it out of the oven and top with sliced green onions.
8.

Cucumber and Tomato Salad

Prep time: 10 minutes
Cook time: 0 minutes
Servings: 4

Ingredients:
- 2 large cucumbers, diced
- 2 cup ofs cherry tomatoes, halved
- 1/4 cup of red onion, thinly sliced
- 2 tbsps chopped fresh parsley
- 2 tbsps chopped fresh dill
- 2 tbsps olive oil

- 1 tbsp red wine vinegar
- Salt and pepper to taste

Instructions:

1. Put the sliced cucumbers, cherry tomatoes, red onion, chopped parsley, and chopped dill in a large mixing basin.
2. A little bowl containing olive oil and red wine vinegar has to be whisked together to make the dressing.Make sure to season with salt and pepper according to your taste.
3. Add the dressing and stir the cucumber and tomato combination until evenly covered.
4. Enjoy right away, or give it a 30-minute chill in the fridge to let the flavors combo.

Baked Parmesan Zucchini Chips

Prep Time: 15 minutes
Cook Time: 25 minutes
Servings: 4

Ingredients:

- 2 medium zucchinis
- 1/2 cup of grated Parmesan cheese
- 1/2 cup of bread crumbs
- 1 teaspoon garlic powder
- 1 teaspoon dried oregano
- Salt and pepper to taste
- Olive oil spray

Instructions:

1. Adjust the oven temperature to 425 °F or 220 °C. To get a baking sheet ready, line it with parchment paper.
2. Step 2: Rinse the zucchini and cut them into thin rounds, approximately 1/4 inch broad.
3. In a small basin, mix together the breadcrumbs, Parmesan cheese, garlic powder, dried oregano, salt, and pepper.
4. Spread out the zucchini slices on the baking sheet you just made. Then, coat each slice equally with the Parmesan mixture.
5. Coat the zucchini slices lightly with olive oil.
6. Step 6: Preheat the oven to a preheated 400°F. Bake for 20 to 25 minutes or until the zucchini chips are crispy and golden.
7. Take it out of the oven and let it a few minutes to cool down before you dig in. These Baked Parmesan Zucchini Chips are absolutely mouthwatering.

Deviled Eggs with a Twist

Prep Time: 20 minutes
Cook Time: 10 minutes
Servings: 6

Ingredients:

- 6 large eggs
- 2 tbsps mayonnaise

* 1 tbsp Dijon mustard
* 1 tbsp pickle relish
* 1/2 teaspoon paprika
* Salt and pepper to taste
* Chopped chives or parsley for garnish (optional)

Instructions:

1. Bring a pot of cold water to a boil and add the eggs. Get the water boiling over medium-high heat.
2. When the water in the saucepan comes to a boil, take it off the heat, cover it, and set the lid for 10 minutes to let the eggs soak.
1. Move the eggs to a basin of ice water and let them cool entirely after 10 minutes. After the eggs have cooled, cut them lengthwise and remove the shells.
3. Gently scoop off the egg yolks and set them aside in a different basin. The egg yolks should be mashed to a smooth consistency using a fork.
2. Step 5: To the mashed yolks, add the mayonnaise, Dijon mustard, pickle relish, paprika, salt, and pepper. Whisk until smooth and creamy.
3. Combine the egg yolks and whites in a pastry bag or spoon and fill the egg whites.
8. For color, sprinkle with more paprika and garnish with chopped chives or parsley if preferred.
4. Deviled eggs should be refrigerated for at least one hour before serving. Savour the delicious Deviled Eggs with a Modern Twist!

Honey Sriracha Roasted Chickpeas

Prep time: 10 minutes
Cook time: 30 minutes
Servings: 4

Ingredients:

* 2 cans of rinsed and drained chickpeas (15 oz each)
* 2 tbsps olive oil
* 2 tbsps honey
* 2 tbsps Sriracha sauce
* 1 teaspoon garlic powder
* 1 teaspoon smoked paprika
* Salt to taste

Instructions:

5. Turn the oven on high heat (400°F, 200°C). Make sure to prepare a baking sheet with foil or parchment paper.
6. To remove any extra moisture, pat the chickpeas dry with paper towels.
7. In a big basin, mix together the honey, olive oil, Sriracha sauce, garlic powder, smoked paprika, and salt. Just mix everything together.
8. Toss the chickpeas in the basin with the honey Sriracha mixture until they are uniformly covered.
9. Arrange the chickpeas on the baking sheet in a single layer.
10. Preheat a baking sheet and roast the chickpeas for 25 to 30 minutes, tossing halfway through, or until they become a golden brown and are crispy.
11. Take it out of the oven and give it a little time to cool down before you dig in. Snack on them or sprinkle them over salads for a crispy treat!

Cheesy Spinach Stuffed Mushrooms

Prep time: 15 minutes
Cook time: 20 minutes
Servings: 6

Ingredients:

- 18 large button mushrooms, stems removed and reserved
- 2 tbsps olive oil
- 2 cloves garlic, minced
- 2 cup ofs fresh spinach, chopped
- 1 cup of shredded mozzarella cheese
- 1/4 cup of grated Parmesan cheese
- Salt and pepper to taste
- Chopped fresh parsley for garnish (optional)

Instructions:

1. Let the oven heat up to 375°F, which is 190°C. Spray or coat a baking dish with olive oil to prevent sticking.
2. Set aside the stems of the mushrooms and finely slice them.
3. Melt the olive oil in a big pan over medium heat. Simmer the chopped stems and minced garlic with the softened mushrooms for a further two or three minutes.
4. Cook the chopped spinach for another two or three minutes, or until it wilts, then add it to the skillet. Make your own seasoning blend using salt and pepper.
5. Take the pan from the heat and give the mixture a little time to cool.
6. Melt the grated Parmesan and shredded mozzarella in a dish with the cooked spinach mixture. Just mix everything together.
7. Gently push down on each mushroom cap to fill it with a dollop of spinach and cheese mixture.
8. Once the baking dish is ready, add the filled mushrooms.
1. To make sure the mushrooms are soft and the cheese is melted and bubbling, bake them in a preheated oven for around fifteen to twenty minutes.
9. When done, take it out of the oven and, if you want, top it with some chopped fresh parsley. As a starter or a side dish, these stuffed mushrooms with spinach and cheese are really mouthwatering.

Roasted Red Pepper and Feta Dip

Prep time: 10 minutes
Cook time: 25 minutes
Servings: 6

Ingredients:

- 2 large red bell peppers
- 1/2 cup of crumbled feta cheese
- 1/4 cup of plain Greek yogurt
- 2 cloves garlic, minced
- 1 tbsp olive oil
- Salt and pepper to taste

- Fresh parsley for garnish (optional)

Instructions:
1. Set oven temperature to 400°F or 200°C. Arrange a baking sheet with parchment paper.
2. Halve the red bell peppers lengthwise and scoop out the seeds and membranes. Put them cut-side down on the baking sheet that you've prepared.
3. Preheat oven to 450 degrees. After 20–25 minutes of roasting, the peppers should have blistered and blackened skins.
4. Move the peppers to a bowl after taking them out of the oven. Place the peppers in the basin and let them cool for ten minutes. After that, cover it with plastic.
5. After the peppers have cooled, remove the burned skin and throw it away.
6. Add the roasted peppers, crumbled feta cheese, Greek yogurt, minced garlic, and olive oil to a food processor. 6. Process until smooth. Beat in the cream until completely combined.
7. Add pepper and salt to taste to the dip.
8. Transfer the dip to a platter, garnish with chopped fresh parsley, and provide with pita bread, crackers, or other vegetables of your choice.

Teriyaki Glazed Edamame

Prep time: 5 minutes
Cook time: 10 minutes
Servings: 4

Ingredients:
- 2 cup ofs frozen edamame, thawed
- 2 tbsps teriyaki sauce
- 1 tbsp sesame oil
- 1 tbsp sesame seeds (optional)
- Season with salt.

Instructions:
1. Heat the sesame oil in a big skillet over medium heat.
1. Toss in the thawed edamame and cook for a couple of minutes in the pan.
2. Disperse the edamame in the teriyaki sauce and toss to combine.
3. Stirring regularly, keep cooking for another 5 to 7 minutes or until the edamame is heated through and the sauce has slightly thickened.
4. Add sesame seeds and salt to taste, if preferred.
5. Step 6: Place the edamame in a serving dish and drizzle with teriyaki glaze. Serve hot for a tasty snack or appetizer.

Bacon-Wrapped Dates

Prep time: 15 minutes
Cook time: 15 minutes
Servings: 12

Ingredients:

- 12 large Medjool dates, pitted
- 6 slices bacon, cut in half
- 24 whole almonds

Instructions:

1. Start by getting your oven ready at 375°F or 190°C. To get a baking sheet ready, line it with parchment paper.
2. Cut a tiny hole in each date and stuff an almond inside.
3. Use a toothpick to secure each date after wrapping it with half a bacon slice.
4. Arrange the dates wrapped in bacon on the baking sheet that you've just prepared.
5. The fifth step is to cook the bacon in a preheated oven until it becomes golden and crispy, which should take approximately 15 minutes.
6. Take it out of the oven and give it a little time to cool down before you dig in. Have fun!

Garlic Herb Roasted Potatoes

Prep time: 10 minutes
Cook time: 30 minutes
Servings: 4

Ingredients:

- 1.5 lbs (680g) baby potatoes, halved
- 2 tbsps olive oil
- 3 cloves garlic, minced
- 1 teaspoon dried thyme
- 1 teaspoon dried rosemary
- Salt and black pepper, to taste
- Fresh parsley, chopped (for garnish)

Instructions:

1. Set oven temperature to 425°F or 220°C. Put parchment paper on a baking pan.
2. Coat the young potatoes in olive oil, chopped garlic, dried thyme, dried rosemary, salt, and black pepper in a big basin. Make sure to toss to coat.
3. In a single layer, spread out the seasoned potatoes on the prepared baking sheet.
6. After the oven is hot, roast the potatoes for 25 to 30 minutes, turning once or until they are soft and browned.
4. When done, take it out of the oven and place it on a platter to serve. As a finishing touch, garnish with some freshly cut parsley.
5. Warm and serve as a tasty accompaniment. Have fun!

Chili Lime Corn on the Cob

Prep time: 10 minutes
Cook time: 20 minutes
Servings: 4

Ingredients:

- 4 ears of corn, husked
- 2 tbsps butter, melted
- 1 lime, juiced and zested
- 1 teaspoon chili powder

- Salt, to taste
- Fresh cilantro, chopped (for garnish, optional)

Instructions:

1. Get your grill ready by heating it up to medium-high heat.
1. The second step is to combine the lime juice, zest, chili powder, salt, and melted butter in a small bowl. Mix well.
2. The next step is to coat the corn kernels uniformly with the spiced butter mixture.
3. Grill the corn for approximately 15 to 20 minutes or until it is slightly browned and soft, turning once or twice.
4. Take the corn from the grill and place it on a plate for serving.
5. If you'd like, you may top it off with chopped cilantro. Warm up and savor!

Cranberry Pecan Chicken Salad Cup ofs

Prep time: 15 minutes
Cook time: 0 minutes
Servings: 12 cup ofs

Ingredients:

- 2 cup ofs cooked chicken, shredded or diced
- 1/2 cup of dried cranberries
- 1/2 cup of pecans, chopped
- 1/3 cup of mayonnaise
- 1/4 cup of plain Greek yogurt
- 1 tbsp Dijon mustard
- 1 tbsp honey
- Salt and pepper, to taste
- 12 mini phyllo pastry shells

Instructions:

1. Throw the cooked chicken, dried cranberries, and pecans into a big basin and stir well.
2. In another little dish, mix the mayonnaise, Greek yogurt, Dijon mustard, honey, salt, and pepper until thoroughly blended.
3. Add the dressing to the chicken mixture and stir until well-covered.
4. Evenly distribute the chicken salad mixture among the miniature phyllo pastry shells and spoon it into each shell.
5. Spoon the filling into the pastry shells; either serve right away or cover and chill until needed.
6. Snack on these tasty Cranberry Pecan Chicken Salad Cup ofs while you wait for your meal to arrive!

Chapter 5: Desserts And Treats

Chocolate Avocado Mousse

Prep time: 10 minutes
Cook time: 0 minutes
Servings: 4

Ingredients:

- 2 ripe avocados
- cocoa powder, 1/4 cup of
- One-fourth cup of of maple syrup or honey
- 1 tsp vanilla extract
- Pinch of salt
- Optional toppings: whipped cream, berries, shaved chocolate

Instructions:

1. After halving the avocados and removing their pits, slice them in half lengthwise and transfer the flesh to a blender or food processor.
2. Put some salt, honey (or maple syrup), vanilla extract, cocoa powder, and the blender on high.
3. The third step is to combine the ingredients until they reach a creamy, smooth consistency, stopping the blender as needed to scrape down the edges.
4. Add additional honey or maple syrup to taste if needed to adjust sweetness.
5. Spoon the mousse into glasses or bowls for serving.
6. Chill in the fridge for half an hour or more before serving.
7. Add berries, whipped cream, or shaved chocolate as garnishes, if preferred.
8. Enjoy when chilled!

Berry Bliss Smoothie Bowl

Prep time: 5 minutes
Cook time: 0 minutes
Servings: 2

Ingredients:

- Blended berries (strawberries, blueberries, raspberries, etc.); 1 cup of
- 1 ripe banana
- 1/2 cup of of Greek yogurt
- one-fourth cup of of almond milk (or milk of your preference)
- one tbsp honey or maple syrup (optional)
- Toppings: granola, sliced fruits, shredded coconut, chia seed

Instructions:

1. In a blender, mix together a variety of berries, a banana, Greek yogurt, almond milk, and, if desired, honey or maple syrup.
2. When blending, add additional almond milk as needed to get the desired consistency. Keep going until you have a creamy, smooth consistency.
3. Divide the smoothie into serving dishes.
4. Sprinkle chia seeds, shredded coconut, sliced fruit, and granola on top.
5. Enjoy your revitalizing Berry Bliss Smoothie Bowl right now by serving it.

Almond Butter Energy Bites

Prep time: 15 minutes

Cook time: 0 minutes
Servings: 12

Ingredients:
- 1 cup of of rolled oats
- 1/2 cup of of almond butter
- One-fourth cup of of honey or maple syrup
- 1/4 cup of of mini chocolate chips
- 1/4 cup of of chopped almonds
- 1 tbsp chia seeds
- 1 tsp vanilla extract
- Pinch of salt

Instructions:
1. In a big bowl, mix together the following ingredients: rolled oats, almond butter, honey or maple syrup, micro chocolate chips, chopped almonds, chia seeds, vanilla essence, and a touch of salt.
2. Make sure to mix everything thoroughly until it's properly combined.
1. Make little balls out of the mixture, each approximately an inch in diameter. Use clean hands to do this.
3. Arrange the energy bites on a parchment-lined baking sheet.
4. Allow to set in the fridge for 30 minutes, minimum, for firmness.
2. Move the energy bites to a container that seals tightly after they are hard. Keep them in the fridge for up to a week.
6. Savor as a healthy and convenient snack

Lemon Poppy Seed Muffins

Prep time: 15 minutes
Cook time: 20 minutes
Servings: 12 muffins

Ingredients:
- 2 cup ofs all-purpose flour
- 1/2 cup of of granulated sugar
- 2 tsp baking powder
- 1/2 tsp baking soda
- 1/4 tsp salt
- Zest of 2 lemons
- 1/4 cup of of lemon juice
- After melting and cooling, use half a cup of of unsalted butter.
- 2 large eggs
- 1 cup of of plain yogurt
- 2 tbsps poppy seeds

Instructions:
1. Get the oven ready by preheating it to 375°F, or 190°C. Prepare the muffin pan's wells by lining them with paper liners or cooking spray.
2. Gather the all-purpose flour, sugar, baking powder, soda, salt, and zest of the lemon into a large mixing basin.
3. Combine the eggs, plain yogurt, melted butter, and lemon juice and mix them together in a separate basin.
4. Add the liquid components to the dry ones and mix gently until just mixed. Make sure not to mix it too much.
5. Evenly distribute the poppy seeds throughout the batter by stirring them in.

6. Pour batter into muffin pans, filling each cup of three-quarters of the way to the top. 6.
7. Preheat oven to 400°F. When a toothpick placed in the middle of a muffin comes out clean, bake for 18 to 20 minutes.
8. Leave the muffins in the pan to cool for 5 minutes after removing from the oven. Once cooled, transfer to a wire rack.
9. After the muffins have cooled, place them in a sealed container and keep them at room temperature for a maximum of three days.
10. No matter the time of day, serve these delicious lemon poppy seed muffins for breakfast or a snack!

Banana Nut Bread

Prep time: 15 minutes
Cook time: 1 hour
Servings: 8 slices

Ingredients:
- 2 ripe bananas, mashed
- 1/3 cup of of melted butter
- 1/2 cup of of granulated sugar
- 1 egg, beaten
- 1 tsp vanilla extract
- 1 tsp baking soda
- Pinch of salt
- 1 1/2 cup of of all-purpose flour
- 1/2 cup of of chopped walnuts

Instructions:
1. Bring the oven temperature up to 350°F, or 175°C. Prepare a 9x5-inch loaf pan with butter.
2. Melt the butter and stir with the mashed bananas in a bowl.
1. Third, combine the banana mixture with the sugar, beaten egg, and vanilla essence. Combine thoroughly.
2. Fourth, combine the salt and baking soda.
5. Mix in the flour gradually until barely incorporated.
6. Mix in the walnuts that have been chopped.
3. Step 7: Transfer the batter to the loaf pan and set it aside to cook.
4. After 60 minutes in a preheated oven, remove the toothpick from the center; it should come out clean.
3. After 10 minutes of chilling in the pan, transfer the banana bread to a wire rack to complete the cooling process.

Coconut Chia Pudding

Prep time: 5 minutes
Cook time: 4 hours
Servings: 2

Ingredients:

- 1/4 cup of of chia seeds
- 1 cup of of coconut milk
- 1 tbsp honey or maple syrup
- 1/2 tsp vanilla extract
- Fresh fruit for serving (optional)

Instructions:

4. First, in a mixing dish, mix together the chia seeds, coconut milk, maple syrup (if using), and vanilla essence.
3. Make sure the chia seeds are dispersed equally by stirring thoroughly.
4. To make the chia seeds thicken, cover the bowl and put it in the fridge for at least four hours or till the next day.
5. To disperse the chia seeds, stir the mixture just before serving.
6. If you'd like, you may top the coconut chia pudding with some fresh fruit before serving.

Pumpkin Spice Cookies

Prep time: 15 minutes
Cook time: 12 minutes
Servings: 24

Ingredients:

- 1 cup of of canned pumpkin puree
- 1/2 cup of of unsalted butter, softened
- 1 cup of of granulated sugar
- 1 large egg
- 1 tsp vanilla extract
- 2 cup of of all-purpose flour
- 1 tsp baking powder
- 1 tsp baking soda
- 1/2 tsp salt
- 1 tsp ground cinnamon
- 1/2 tsp ground nutmeg
- 1/4 tsp ground cloves
- 1/4 tsp ground ginger
- 1 cup of of white chocolate chips (optional)

Instructions:

1. It all starts with getting the oven up to 350 degrees Fahrenheit (175 degrees Celsius) and lining a baking sheet with parchment paper.
2. Whip the granulated sugar and softened butter in a large bowl until the mixture is light and fluffy.
3. Third, while the cream is still beating, add the pumpkin puree, egg, and vanilla essence. Whisk until well blended.
4. Toss the flour, baking soda, salt, cinnamon, nutmeg, ginger, and cloves in a separate basin.
5. To make the cookie dough, slowly combine the dry components with the liquid ones while mixing constantly.
6. If desired, stir in the white chocolate chips.
7. Spread out the dough on the baking sheet and drop tbsp fulls into it, leaving approximately 2 inches of space between each.
8. Eight put it in the preheated oven and bake for ten to twelve minutes, or until the sides start to become golden.

9. Set the cookies on a wire rack to cool fully after removing them from the baking sheet, which should take a few minutes.
10. Pumpkin Spice Cookies are excellent.

Apple Cinnamon Oat Bars

Prep time: 15 minutes
Cook time: 25 minutes
Servings: Makes 12 bars

Ingredients:

- 2 cup ofs of old-fashioned oats
- 1 cup of of all-purpose flour
- 1/2 cup of of brown sugar, packed
- 1/2 tsp baking powder
- 1/4 tsp salt
- 1 tsp ground cinnamon
- 1/2 cup of of unsalted butter, melted
- 2 medium apples, peeled, cored, and diced
- 1 tbsp lemon juice
- 2 tbsps granulated sugar

Instructions:

1. First, oil or line an 8x8-inch baking sheet with parchment paper and set oven temperature to 350°F, or 175°C.
2. Put the cinnamon, brown sugar, oats, flour, baking powder, and salt into a big basin.
3. Once the mixture is crumbly and uniformly moistened, pour in the melted butter and whisk.
4. Scatter half of the oat mixture evenly over the bottom of the baking pan that you just made.
5. In another bowl, combine the granulated sugar, lemon juice, and chopped apples. Toss to coat.
6. Evenly distribute the apple mixture over the oats that have been layered in the baking pan.
7. Gently push down on the apples and sprinkle the remaining oat mixture over top.
8. Preheat the oven to 375°F and bake for 25 to 30 minutes, or until the apples are soft and the top is browned.
9. Let the bars cool for 15 minutes in the pan before cutting them into squares.
10. Apple Cinnamon Oat Bars are delicious, warm, or served at room temperature.

Peanut Butter Chocolate Chip Cookies

Prep time: 15 minutes
Cook time: 10 minutes
Servings: 24

Ingredients:

- 1 cup of of peanut butter
- 1 cup of of granulated sugar
- 1 large egg
- 1 tsp vanilla extract
- 1/2 cup of of chocolate chips

Instructions:

1. Mix with salt and pepper and bake at 350 degrees F (that's 175 degrees C) on a lined baking sheet.
2. In a big bowl, combine the peanut butter, sugar, egg, and vanilla essence. Stir to combine. Incorporate all components and blend until homogeneous.
3. Gently incorporate the chocolate chips into the dough, making sure they are spread equally.
4. Space the dough spheres on the prepared baking sheet approximately 2 inches apart. Use a tbsp or cookie scoop to put the dough balls onto the sheet.
5. Use a fork to gently flatten each ball, creating a crisscross pattern on top.
6. To make the cookies golden brown on the edges, place them in the prepared oven and bake for 10 to 12 minutes.
7. Move the cookies from the baking sheet to a wire rack to cool completely after a few minutes.
8. Dip those tasty Peanut Butter Chocolate Chip Cookies into some deliciousness!

Mango Coconut Sorbet

Prep time: 10 minutes
Cook time: 0 minutes
Servings: 4

Ingredients:
- 2 ripe mangoes, peeled and chopped
- 1/2 cup of of coconut milk
- 2 tbsps honey or agave syrup (optional, adjust to taste)
- 1 tbsp lime juice
- Shredded coconut and mint leaves for garnish (optional)

Instructions:
1. Throw the mango chunks, coconut milk, honey (if using), and lime juice into a food processor or blender.
1. Be sure to scrape down the sides of the blender as needed as you blend until the mixture is smooth and creamy.
2. If you find that the combination is too sweet, add additional honey or agave syrup to taste.
3. Cover the mixture with plastic wrap and move it to a shallow dish or container.
4. Once the sorbet has been set, put the container in the freezer for at least four hours.
5. After the sorbet has frozen, take it out of the freezer and allow it to remain at room temperature for a short while to become somewhat softer.
6. Scoop the sorbet into dishes using an ice cream scoop.
7. If you like, you may top it up with some shredded coconut and mint leaves.
8. Pour into glasses and savor the cool mango coconut sorbet right away!

Espresso Protein Brownies

Prep time: 15 minutes
Cook time: 25 minutes
Servings: 12

Ingredients:

- 1 cup of of almond flour
- 1/4 cup of of cocoa powder
- 1/4 cup of of chocolate protein powder
- 1/2 cup of of coconut sugar
- 2 tbsps espresso powder
- 1/2 tsp baking powder
- 1/4 tsp salt
- 1/2 cup of of almond milk
- 1/4 cup of of melted coconut oil
- 2 eggs
- 1 tsp vanilla extract
- 1/4 cup of of dark chocolate chips

Instructions:

1. Peel off the parchment paper and prepare an 8-by-8-inch baking sheet. Turn the oven on high heat (350°F, 175°C).
1. Almond flour, cocoa powder, protein powder, coconut sugar, espresso powder, baking powder, and salt should all be whisked together in a big basin.
2. Mix the almond milk, eggs, melted coconut oil, and vanilla extract in a separate bowl.
3. Gradually mix the dry components with the wet ones.
4. Gently incorporate the dark chocolate chunks.
5. After you put aside the baking pan, evenly spread the batter into it.
6. To test whether it's done, stick a toothpick into the middle and bake for 25 minutes.
7. Let the brownies cool entirely before cutting them into serving pieces.

Raspberry Almond Thumbprint Cookies

Prep time: 20 minutes
Cook time: 12 minutes
Servings: 24

Ingredients:

- 1 cup of of almond flour
- 1/4 cup of of coconut flour
- 1/4 cup of of coconut sugar
- 1/4 tsp salt
- 1/4 cup of of coconut oil, melted
- 1 egg
- 1 tsp almond extract
- 1/4 cup of of raspberry jam

Instructions:

1. Bake at 350 degrees Fahrenheit (175 degrees Celsius) using a parchment-lined baking sheet.
2. Blend together the flours of almonds, coconuts, sugar from coconuts, and salt in a big basin.
1. Third, make a dough by mixing in the egg, almond essence, and melted coconut oil.
3. On the baking sheet that has been prepared, roll the dough into 1-inch balls.
4. Make a well in the middle of each biscuit using your thumb or the back of a spoon.
5. Spoon raspberry jam into each depression.
6. Put the cookies in the oven and bake for 12 minutes or until they are just brown and firm.
7. Take the cookies from the baking pan after 5 minutes and set them on a wire rack to cool completely.

Pineapple Upside-Down Cake Bites

Prep time: 15 minutes
Cook time: 20 minutes
Servings: 12

Ingredients:
- 1 cup of of almond flour
- 1/4 cup of of coconut flour
- 1/4 cup of of coconut sugar
- 1/2 tsp baking powder
- 1/4 tsp salt
- 1/4 cup of of melted coconut oil
- 1/4 cup of of unsweetened almond milk
- 2 eggs
- 1 tsp vanilla extract
- 1 cup of of diced pineapple, drained
- 1/4 cup of of maraschino cherries, drained and halved

Instructions:
1. To begin, grease a small muffin tray and heat the oven to 350 degrees Fahrenheit or 175°C.
2. Step 2: In a big basin, mix the flours of almonds, coconuts, sugar, baking soda, and salt.
3. Mix in almond milk, eggs, vanilla essence, and melted coconut oil until well blended.
4. Fill each muffin cup of with a few sliced pineapple slices and a half cherry.
5. Fill up each cup of three-quarters of the way to the top with cake batter, then spoon it over the pineapple and cherry.
6. When a toothpick inserted in the center comes out clean and the sides have just browned, remove from the oven and continue baking for another 20 minutes.
7. Once 5 minutes have passed, carefully remove the cake pieces from the muffin tray and place them on a wire rack to cool completely.

Blueberry Lemon Loaf

Prep time: 15 minutes
Cook time: 50 minutes
Servings: 8 slices

Ingredients:

- 1½ cup of of all-purpose flour
- 1 tsp baking powder
- ½ tsp baking soda
- ¼ tsp salt
- ½ cup of of unsalted butter softened
- 1 cup of of granulated sugar
- 2 large eggs
- 1 tsp vanilla extract
- Zest of 1 lemon
- ⅓ cup of of fresh lemon juice
- ½ cup of of buttermilk
- 1 cup of of fresh blueberries

Instructions:

1. Bring the oven temperature up to 350°F, or 175°C. Pat a loaf pan that measures 9 by 5 inches with flour and grease.
1. Second, combine the flour, baking soda, salt, baking powder, and baking powder in a medium basin. Whisk to combine. Remove off the table.
2. Whip the sugar and softened butter in a large basin until the mixture is light and airy.
3. Add the eggs one by one while beating, then add the vanilla essence, zest, and juice of the lemons.
4. Gradually, alternating between the wet and dry components, slowly add them to the wet mixture. Start with the dry ingredients and conclude with the buttermilk. Blend only until barely mixed.
5. Add the fresh blueberries, folding gently so as not to crush them.
6. Seven, once the loaf pan has been heated, pour in the batter and smooth the top with a spatula.
7. To test whether it's ready, stick a toothpick into the middle and bake for 45 to 50 minutes or until it comes out clean.
8. Transfer the loaf to a wire rack to complete cooling after 10 minutes of cooling in the pan.

Vanilla Bean Rice Pudding

Prep time: 5 minutes
Cook time: 30 minutes
Servings: 4

Ingredients:

- ½ cup of of Arborio rice
- 3 cup ofs of whole milk
- about half a cup of of sugar that has been ground into fine powder
- Use 1 teaspoon of vanilla essence or 1 split vanilla bean with the seeds removed.
- Pinch of salt
- Ground cinnamon, for garnish (optional)

Instructions:

1. A medium-sized saucepan should be used to combine the Arborio rice, whole milk, sugar, vanilla bean seeds, and salt.
2. Second, bring to a simmer over medium heat, stirring once or twice, for two minutes.
3. Simmer, covered, over low heat for 25-30 minutes, or until rice is cooked through and pudding has thickened, stirring once in a while.
4. Take the pan from the stove and, if used, throw away the pod of the vanilla bean.
5. Garnish with a sprinkling of ground cinnamon, if preferred, and serve the rice pudding warm or cold.

Strawberry Shortcake Cup of of

Prep time: 20 minutes
Cook time: 15 minutes
Servings: 6

Ingredients:

- 1½ cup of of all-purpose flour
- ¼ cup of of granulated sugar
- 1½ tsp baking powder
- ¼ tsp salt
- 6 tbsps cold unsalted butter, cut into small pieces
- ½ cup of of milk
- 1 tsp vanilla extract
- 2 cup of of sliced strawberries
- 2 tbsps granulated sugar
- Whipped cream for serving

Instructions:

1. Set oven temperature to 400°F, or 200°C. Make sure to grease or line a muffin pan with paper liners.
2. Second, mix the flour, sugar, baking soda, and salt in a big basin.
3. Incorporate the chilled butter into the mixture by chopping it with a pastry blender or two knives until it resembles coarse crumbs.
4. Fourth, combine the milk and vanilla essence in a different basin. When a dough develops, gradually add the milk mixture while stirring in the flour mixture.
5. Roll out the dough and press it evenly into the bottom and up the sides of each muffin cup of.
6. Combine the granulated sugar and cut strawberries in a small dish. Fill the middle of each dough cup of with strawberries.
7. Once the oven is hot, place the shortcake cup ofs inside and cook for 12–15 minutes or until they start to turn a golden brown color.
8. Eight, after a few minutes, take the muffin tray out of the oven and set the shortcake cup ofs on a wire rack to cool completely.
9. Spoon whipped cream on top of each cup of of shortcake.

Carrot Cake Energy Balls

Prep time: 15 minutes
Cook time: 0 minutes
Servings: 12

Ingredients:

- 1 cup of of rolled oats
- 1/2 cup of of shredded carrots
- 1/4 cup of of chopped walnuts
- 1/4 cup of of raisins
- 2 tbsps maple syrup
- 1 tbsp almond butter
- 1 tsp ground cinnamon
- 1/2 tsp ground nutmeg
- 1/4 tsp ground ginger
- Pinch of salt
- Optional: shredded coconut for rolling

Instructions:

1. First, in a food processor, mix together the following ingredients: rolled oats, chopped walnuts, raisins, maple syrup, almond butter, cinnamon, ginger, nutmeg, and a touch of salt.
2. Pulse the ingredients until they are thoroughly mixed and start to resemble dough.
3. Form little balls out of the mixture, each approximately an inch in diameter.
4. For an additional taste boost, you can opt to roll the energy balls in shredded coconut.
5. Chill the energy balls in the fridge for half an hour before you eat them.
6. Savor as a nutritious and tasty snack!

Chocolate Covered Strawberries

Prep time: 10 minutes
Cook time: 5 minutes
Servings: 4

Ingredients:

- Fresh strawberries
- 1 cup of of semi-sweet chocolate chips
- 1 tbsp coconut oil

Instructions:

1. First, give the strawberries a quick rinse and then dry them off with paper towels.
2. Blend the chocolate chips and coconut oil in a microwave-safe bowl.
3. Melt and smooth the chocolate in the microwave in 30-second intervals, stirring every 30 seconds.
4. Spread the melted chocolate on each strawberry by dipping them all the way through.
5. Put the strawberries on a parchment-lined baking sheet.
6. Let the chocolate firm in the fridge for approximately fifteen to twenty minutes.
7. Present this mouth-watering dessert and savor it!

Peach Cobbler Parfait

Prep time: 10 minutes
Cook time: 0 minutes
Servings: 2-4

Ingredients:

- 2 cup ofs of diced peaches
- 1 cup of of Greek yogurt
- 1/2 cup of of granola
- 2 tbsps honey
- 1/2 tsp ground cinnamon
- Whipped cream (optional)

Instructions:

1. Coat the chopped peaches well with the honey and ground cinnamon in a bowl.
2. Arrange the Greek yogurt, chopped peach combination, and granola in serving plates or glasses in that order.
3. Keep piling on the layers until all of the bowls or glasses are full.
1. Optional: garnish with whipped cream.
2. Enjoy this delicious peach cobbler-inspired parfait right away by serving it hot.

Key Lime Pie Bites

Prep time: 20 minutes
Cook time: 0 minutes
Servings: 12

Ingredients:

- 1 cup of of almond flour
- 1/4 cup of of coconut flour
- 1/4 cup of of maple syrup
- 1/4 cup of of coconut oil, melted
- Zest and juice of 2 limes
- 1 tsp vanilla extract
- Pinch of salt
- Shredded coconut (optional for rolling)

Instructions:

1. A touch of salt, lime zest, lime juice, almond flour, coconut flour, maple syrup, heated coconut oil, and a mixing bowl are the ingredients you need. Stir until a cohesive dough is formed.
2. Pat the dough into little balls, each approximately one inch in size.
3. If you want to add some more texture and taste, you may optionally roll the balls in shredded coconut.
4. Arrange the bite-sized key lime pie on a parchment-lined baking sheet.
5. Chill for half an hour or more prior to consumption.
6. Savor these tasty bits of key lime pie, which are both refreshing and taste

<u>Chapter 6: Beverages</u>

Tropical Sunrise Smoothie

Prep time: 5 minutes
Cook time: 0 minutes
Servings: 2

Ingredients:

- 1 ripe banana
- 1 cup of of fresh pineapple chunks
- 1/2 cup of of mango chunks
- 1/2 cup of of orange juice
- 1/2 cup of of coconut water
- 1/2 cup of of Greek yogurt (optional)
- Ice cubes (optional)

Instructions:

1. Slice the banana lengthwise after peeling it.
2. Blend the pineapple, mango, banana, orange juice, and coconut water until smooth.
3. If you want it extra creamy, add Greek yogurt.
4. Whip everything together until it's completely combined.
5. To make it colder, juice some ice cubes and blend them with the smoothie ingredients.
6. Fill glasses with smoothie mixture and serve right away.
7. Suck on that tropical sunrise smoothie! It's so refreshing!

Berry Blast Refreshment

Prep time: 5 minutes
Cook time: 0 minutes
Servings: 2

Ingredients:

- 1 cup of of a variety of berries, including raspberries, blueberries, and strawberries.
- 1/2 cup of of vegan or non-dairy yogurt
- Half a cup of of almond milk (or milk of your preference, really)
- 1 tbsp honey (optional)
- Ice cubes (optional)

Instructions:

1. Rinse the mixed berries and cut off the stems.
2. Add the almond milk, fruit, yogurt, and honey (if desired) to a blender.
3. Process until the mixture is completely smooth.
4. Throw in a few ice cubes and puree the mixture for a chillier beverage.
5. Add additional honey to taste if you want it sweeter. 6. Taste again.
6. Fill glasses with Berry Blast Refreshment and serve right away.
7. Add fresh berries as a garnish if you want.
8. Savour the tasty and healthy Berry Blast Refreshment!

Minty Mojito Cooler

Prep time: 10 minutes
Cook time: 0 minutes
Servings: 2

Ingredients:

- 10 fresh mint leaves
- 1 lime, sliced
- 2 tbsps sugar
- Ice cubes
- 1 cup of of club soda
- 2 oz white rum (optional)
- Lime wedges and mint sprigs for garnish

Instructions:

1. Add the sugar, lime slices, and mint leaves to a strong glass and mix until aromatic.
2. Second, put ice cubes into the glass.
3. Add the club soda to the ice and mix well.
4. If you'd like, you may also add white rum.
5. Add mint leaves and lime wedges as garnishes.
6. Enjoy your revitalizing Minty Mojito Cooler right now by serving it.

Citrus Zing Infusion

Prep time: 5 minutes
Cook time: 0 minutes
Servings: 2

Ingredients:

- 1 orange, sliced
- 1 lemon, sliced
- 1 lime, sliced
- 2 tbsps honey
- Ice cubes
- 2 cup ofs of water
- Orange, lemon, and lime slices for garnish

Instructions:

1. Slice the orange, lemon, and lime and put them in a pitcher.
2. Pour the honey and lightly crush the fruit to extract its juices.
3. Add ice cubes to the pitcher.
4. Add water to the ice and mix well.
5. Give the infusion a few minutes to settle so the flavors can combine.
6. Transfer to serving glasses and, if preferred, top with extra slices of citrus.
7. Your Citrus Zing Infusion is ready to enjoy when served cold.

Iced Caramel Macchiato:

Prep time: 5 minutes
Cook time: 0 minutes
Servings: 1

Ingredients:

- 1 shot of espresso
- 1 cup of of milk
- 2 tbsps of caramel syrup
- Ice cubes

Instructions:

1. Allow a shot of espresso to cool down after brewing.
2. To make a glass, add ice cubes.
3. Drizzle the ice with the caramel syrup.
4. Gradually drizzle the milk over the syrup and ice.
5. Top with the cooled espresso.
6. Before you savor your Iced Caramel Macchiato, carefully stir it.

Pineapple Paradise Punch:

Prep time: 10 minutes
Cook time: 0 minutes
Servings: 4

Ingredients:

- 2 cup ofs of pineapple juice
- 1 cup of of orange juice
- 1 cup of of coconut water
- 1 cup of of sparkling water
- Pineapple slices and mint leaves for garnish
- Ice cubes

Instructions:

1. The pineapple juice, orange juice, sparkling water, and coconut water should be combined in a big pitcher.
2. Pour ice cubes into small glasses.
3. Slowly pour the punch over the ice
4. Add pineapple slices and mint leaves as garnishes. Enjoy your Pineapple Paradise Punch when served cold.

Green Goddess Detox Drink:

Prep time: 5 minutes
Cook time: 0 minutes
Servings: 2

Ingredients:

- 2 cup ofs of spinach
- 1 cucumber, peeled and chopped
- 1 green apple, cored and chopped
- 1 lemon, juiced
- 1 tbsp of honey (optional)
- Ice cubes

Instructions:

1. In a blender, combine the spinach, cucumber, green apple, and lemon juice. Blend until smooth.
2. If desired, add honey for sweetness and blend again.
3. Fill glasses with ice cubes.
4. Pour the Green Goddess detox drink over the ice.
5. Stir gently and enjoy your refreshing and healthy detox drink!

Creamy Coconut Frappe

Prep time: 5 minutes
Cook time: 0 minutes
Servings: 2

Ingredients:

- 1 cup of of coconut milk
- 1 cup of of ice cubes
- 2 tbsps honey or maple syrup
- 1/2 tsp vanilla extract
- Whipped cream (optional)
- Shredded coconut, for garnish (optional)

Instructions:

1. Put the ice cubes, coconut milk, honey (or maple syrup), and vanilla essence into a blender.
2. Whip until fully combined and creamy.
1. Third, transfer to serving glasses and garnish with shredded coconut and whipped cream, if you like.
2. Enjoy right away after serving!

Energizing Matcha Latte

Prep time: 5 minutes
Cook time: 5 minutes
Servings: 1

Ingredients:

- 1 tsp matcha powder
- 1 tbsp hot water
- 1 cup of of milk (any type)
- 1 tbsp honey or sweetener of choice
- Ice cubes (optional)

Instructions:

1. After the water has been heated, whisk in the matcha powder until a smooth consistency is achieved.
2. Make sure the milk is heated, but not boiling, in a saucepan over medium heat.
3. Take the milk from the heat and whisk in the matcha and honey until creamy.

1. For a chilled variation, you may pour the latte over ice cubes if you choose.
2. Enjoy the revitalizing matcha latte right away by serving it.

Watermelon Mint Cooler

Prep time: 10 minutes
Cook time: 0 minutes
Servings: 2

Ingredients:

- 2 cup ofs of diced watermelon
- 1/4 cup of of fresh mint leaves
- 1 tbsp honey or agave syrup
- 1 tbsp lime juice
- 1 cup of of cold water
- Ice cubes
- Mint sprigs and watermelon slices for garnish (optional)

Instructions:

1. In a blender, combine the diced watermelon, fresh mint leaves, honey or agave syrup, lime juice, and cold water.
2. Blend until smooth.
3. Empty the mixture of any pulp by passing it through a fine-mesh sieve.
4. Pour the watermelon mixture into glasses filled with ice cubes.
5. Garnish with mint sprigs and watermelon slices if desired.
6. Serve immediately and enjoy the refreshing watermelon mint cooler!

Blueberry Lavender Lemonade

Prep time: 10 minutes
Cook time: 0 minutes
Servings: 4

Ingredients:

- 1 cup of of fresh blueberries
- 1/4 cup of of dried lavender buds
- 1 cup of of fresh lemon juice
- 1/2 cup of of honey or sugar
- 4 cup ofs of cold water
- Cubes of ice
- Decorative elements like lemon wedges and fresh lavender sprigs are welcome additions.

Instructions:

1. Blueberries, dried lavender buds, and a cup of of water should be mixed in a small saucepan. 5. After 5 minutes of simmering over medium heat, remove the flame. Leave it on the hob until it cools entirely.
2. Press down on the particles to extract as much liquid as possible as you strain the blueberry-lavender combination through a fine mesh sieve into a large pitcher.
3. Three cup ofs of cold water, together with the fresh lemon juice, honey, or sugar, should be added to the pitcher. Dissolve the sweetener by stirring.
4. In order to cool the lemonade, place it in the refrigerator for at least 1 hour.
5. Pour the lemonade with blueberries and lavender over ice and serve. Toss in some lemon slices and fresh lavender sprigs for garnish if you want. Savour it!

Spiced Chai Tea Latte

Prep time: 5 minutes
Cook time: 5 minutes
Servings: 2

Ingredients:

- 2 cup ofs of water
- 2 black tea bags
- 1 cinnamon stick
- 4 whole cloves
- 4 cardamom pods, lightly crushed
- 1-inch piece of fresh ginger, thinly sliced
- 2 cup ofs of milk (any type - dairy or non-dairy)
- 2 tbsps honey or sugar (adjust to taste)
- Ground cinnamon for garnish (optional)

Instructions:

1. Boil some water in a small pot. You may garnish it with sliced ginger, cinnamon sticks, cloves, cardamom pods, and black tea bags.
2. Bring the tea to a simmer over low heat for 5 minutes to let the spices infuse.
3. Keep the milk from boiling by bringing it to a simmer in a separate pot over medium heat.
4. Take the spiced tea mixture off the heat and throw away the tea bags.
5. Add the scalding milk to the spiced tea and mix well.
1. Step 6: Sweeten the chai latte according to your liking by adding honey or sugar.
6. Pour the chai latte into individual glasses after straining through a fine mesh filter.
7. If you want to garnish it, you may sprinkle powdered cinnamon on top. Make a piping hot cup of of spiced chai tea and sip on it until it warms you up

Raspberry Lemon Sparkler

Prep time: 5 minutes

Cook time: 0 minutes
Servings: 2

Ingredients:

- 1 cup of of fresh raspberries
- 2 tbsps lemon juice
- 2 tbsps honey
- 2 cup ofs of sparkling water
- Ice cubes
- Lemon slices and fresh raspberries for garnish

Instructions:

1. In a blender, combine the fresh raspberries, lemon juice, and honey. Blend until smooth.
2. Strain the raspberry mixture through a fine mesh sieve to remove the seeds.
3. Fill two glasses with ice cubes.
4. Divide the strained raspberry mixture evenly between the glasses.
5. Top each glass with 1 cup of of sparkling water.
6. Stir gently to combine.
7. Garnish with lemon slices and fresh raspberries.
8. Serve immediately and enjoy!

Honeydew Basil Refresher

Prep time: 10 minutes
Cook time: 0 minutes
Servings: 2

Ingredients:

- 2 cup of of cubed honeydew melon
- 1/4 cup of of fresh basil leaves
- 2 tbsps lime juice
- 1 tbsp honey
- 2 cup ofs of coconut water
- Ice cubes
- Honeydew melon balls and fresh basil leaves for garnish

Instructions:

1. In a blender, combine the cubed honeydew melon, fresh basil leaves, lime juice, and honey. Blend until smooth.
2. Strain the honeydew mixture through a fine mesh sieve to remove any pulp.
3. Fill two glasses with ice cubes.
4. Divide the strained honeydew mixture evenly between the glasses.
5. Top each glass with 1 cup of of coconut water.
6. Stir gently to combine.
7. Garnish with honeydew melon balls and fresh basil leaves.
8. Serve immediately and enjoy!

Peachy Keen Iced Tea

Prep time: 5 minutes
Cook time: 5 minutes
Servings: 2

Ingredients:

- 2 cup ofs of brewed peach tea, chilled
- 1/2 cup of of peach nectar
- 1 tbsp lemon juice
- 2 tsp honey (optional)
- Ice cubes
- Peach slices and fresh mint leaves for garnish

Instructions:

1. In a pitcher, combine the chilled brewed peach tea, peach nectar, lemon juice, and honey (if using). Stir until well combined.
2. Fill two glasses with ice cubes.
3. Divide the peach tea mixture evenly between the glasses.
4. Garnish each glass with peach slices and fresh mint leaves.
5. Serve immediately and enjoy!

Golden Turmeric Elixir

Prep time: 5 minutes
Cook time: 5 minutes
Servings: 2

Ingredients:

- 2 cup ofs of almond milk
- 1 tsp ground turmeric
- 1/2 tsp ground ginger
- 1/4 tsp ground cinnamon
- 1 tbsp honey or maple syrup
- Ground black pepper (to improve turmeric's bioavailability)
- Optional: Dash of cayenne pepper for a spicy kick

Instructions:

1. Be cautious not to boil the almond milk when you heat it in a small pot over medium heat.
1. After that, add the ground ginger, cinnamon, honey (or maple syrup), and black pepper and whisk until everything is incorporated.
2. Simmer, stirring periodically, for three to five minutes.
3. Take the turmeric elixir from the stove and pour it into glasses.
4. For an additional kick, you may optionally sprinkle a little cayenne pepper.
5. Simmer till warm, then savor the calming and nourishing effects of this elixir.

Chocolate Banana Smoothie

Prep time: 5 minutes
Cook time: 0 minutes
Servings: 2

Ingredients:

- 2 ripe bananas, peeled and sliced
- 1 cup of of milk (almond or otherwise)
- 2 tbsps cocoa powder
- 1 tbsp honey or maple syrup (optional, depending on sweetness preference)
- 1/2 tsp vanilla extract
- 1 cup of of ice cubes

Instructions:

1. In a blender, combine the sliced bananas, almond milk, chocolate powder, vanilla extract, honey or maple syrup (if desired), and ice cubes.
2. With occasional scraping of the blender's sides, mix on high speed until a smooth and creamy consistency is achieved.
3. If you want it sweeter, add extra maple syrup or honey to taste.
4. Fill up each glass with the chocolate banana smoothie.
5. If desired, top with chopped bananas or chocolate powder.
1. Make this guilt-free chocolate dessert right now and savor every bite!

Cranberry Orange Spritzer

Prep time: 5 minutes
Cook time: 0 minutes
Servings: 2

Ingredients:

- 1 cup of of cranberry juice
- 1 cup of of orange juice
- 1 cup of of sparkling water
- Ice cubes
- Orange slices for garnish (optional)

Instructions:

1. In a pitcher, combine cranberry juice, orange juice, and sparkling water.
2. Stir well to mix.
3. Fill serving glasses with ice cubes.
4. Pour the spritzer over the ice.
5. Garnish with orange slices, if desired.
6. Serve immediately and enjoy!

Vanilla Almond Milkshake

Prep time: 5 minutes
Cook time: 0 minutes
Servings: 2

Ingredients:

- 2 cup ofs of vanilla ice cream
- 1 cup of of almond milk

- 1 tsp vanilla extract
- 2 tbsps sliced almonds (optional)
- Whipped cream for topping (optional)
- Maraschino cherry for garnish (optional)

Instructions:

1. The first step is to incorporate almond milk, vanilla extract, and vanilla ice cream.
2. Process until a creamy consistency is achieved.
3. Third, if you'd like, you may add sliced almonds and pulse the blender a few times to combine.
4. Transfer the milkshake to individual glasses for serving.
5. If you'd like, garnish with whipped cream and a maraschino cherry.
6. Enjoy your tasty vanilla almond milkshake right away by serving it right now.

Pomegranate Ginger Fizz

Prep time: 10 minutes
Cook time: 0 minutes
Servings: 2

Ingredients:

- 1 cup of of pomegranate juice
- 1/2 cup of of ginger ale
- 1/4 cup of of sparkling water
- 2 tbsps fresh lime juice
- Ice cubes
- Lime slices for garnish
- Fresh mint leaves, for garnish

Instructions:

1. Measure out the pomegranate juice, ginger ale, sparkling water, and fresh lime juice into a pitcher.
2. Pour in all the ingredients and stir until fully combined.
3. Now, add ice cubes to two glasses.
4. Pour the pomegranate ginger mixture into each glass in an equal distribution.
5. Top off each glass with a lime wedge and a sprig of mint.
6. Serve right away and enjoy the invigorating Pomegranate Ginger Fizz!

Chapter 7: Soups And Salads

Garden Fresh Salad with Balsamic Vinaigrette

Prep time: 10 minutes
Cook time: 0 minutes
Servings: 4

Ingredients:

- 6 cup ofs of mixed salad greens (such as lettuce, spinach, and arugula)
- 1 cup of of cherry tomatoes, halved
- 1 cucumber, sliced
- 1/2 red onion, thinly sliced
- 1/4 cup of of crumbled feta cheese
- 1/4 cup of of chopped walnuts (optional)

Instructions:

1. Season with the dressing: In a little bowl, make a thorough mixture of the balsamic vinegar, lemon juice, salt, and pepper. Remove the table.
2. The rest of the ingredients should be mixed together in a big salad bowl.
3. After adding the dressing, mix the salad to combine.

Creamy Tomato Basil Soup

Prep Time: 10 minutes
Cook Time: 25 minutes
Servings: 4

Ingredients:

- 2 tbsps olive oil
- 1 onion, chopped
- 2 cloves garlic, minced
- 2 (14.5 oz) cans diced tomatoes
- 2 cup ofs of vegetable broth
- Fresh basil, freshly chopped, about 1/4 cup of
- 1/2 cup of of heavy cream
- Salt and pepper to taste
- Fresh basil leaves for garnish (optional)

Instructions:

1. Melt the olive oil in a big saucepan over medium heat. Saute for about 5 minutes, or until the onion and garlic are cooked, after which add the minced garlic.
2. Put the chopped tomatoes and their juices into the saucepan along with the vegetable broth. Cook, covered, at a low simmer for fifteen minutes.
3. Smooth up the soup by blending it with an immersion blender or by pouring the ingredients into a blender.
4. Toss in the heavy cream and chopped basil leaves; reheat the soup if necessary. To taste, season with salt and pepper.
5. Heat through, stirring periodically, for another 5 minutes.
1. Serve hot, ladle into dishes, and top with fresh basil leaves, if preferred.
6. Soup with creamy tomato basil is ready to be enjoyed!

Southwest Quinoa Salad with Lime Dressing

Prep time: 15 minutes
Cook time: 20 minutes
Servings: 4

Ingredients:

- 1 cup of of quinoa
- 1 ½ cup ofs of water
- 15 ozs (one can) of rinsed and drained black beans
- 1 cup of kernels of corn, either fresh or frozen
- 1 chopped red bell pepper
- 1 avocado, diced
- ¼ cup of of chopped fresh cilantro
- Juice of 2 limes
- 2 tbsps olive oil
- 1 tsp ground cumin
- Salt and pepper to taste

Instructions:

1. Before cooking, give the quinoa a good rinsing in cold water.
2. Boil the water in a medium pot. Once the water has been absorbed and the quinoa has cooked, cover and simmer for 15-20 minutes over low heat or until the quinoa is done.
3. Add the cooked quinoa, black beans, corn, red pepper, avocado, and cilantro to a big bowl. Stir to blend.
4. A small bowl containing lime juice, olive oil, ground cumin, salt, and pepper is used to make the dressing.
5. Add the dressing and mix the salad until evenly distributed.
6. Enjoy it right away, or keep it in the fridge until you're ready to dig in.

Butternut Squash Soup with Apple and Sage

Prep time: 15 minutes
Cook time: 30 minutes
Servings: 6

Ingredients:

- 1 butternut squash, each medium, peeled, seeded, and chopped
- 1 tbsp olive oil
- 1 onion, diced
- 2 cloves garlic, minced
- 1 apple, peeled, cored, and diced
- 4 cup ofs of vegetable broth
- ½ tsp dried sage
- Salt and pepper to taste
- ¼ cup of of heavy cream (optional)
- Fresh sage leaves for garnish (optional)

Instructions:

1. Turn the olive oil to medium heat in a big saucepan. Once the garlic and onion are diced, sauté for about 5 minutes or until softer.
2. Cook, stirring occasionally, for another 5 minutes after adding the chopped apple and butternut squash.
3. Put the sage essence and vegetable stock into the mixture. Simmer, covered, for 20–25 minutes (or until reduced in volume), after which bring to a boil.
4. Blend the soup until it's completely smooth, either using an immersion blender or dividing it into batches and transferring it to a blender.
5. Five, season with salt and pepper to taste. Incorporate the heavy cream into the soup by whisking until combined.
6. Top with fresh sage leaves and serve hot.

Greek Salad with Feta and Kalamata Olives

Prep time: 15 minutes
Cook time: 0 minutes
Servings: 4

Ingredients:

- 4 cup ofs of chopped romaine lettuce
- 1 cucumber, diced
- 1 cup of of cherry tomatoes, halved
- 1/2 red onion, thinly sliced
- 1/2 cup of of crumbled feta cheese
- 1/4 cup of of Kalamata olives
- Extra virgin olive oil, 1/4 cup of
- 2 tbsps red wine vinegar
- 1 tsp dried oregano
- Salt and pepper to taste

Instructions:

1. In a big salad bowl, mix together the romaine lettuce, cucumber, cherry tomatoes, and thinly sliced red onion. Blend and toss to blend.
2. Toss in the Kalamata olives and crumbled feta cheese.
3. On the third step, make the dressing by mixing together the oregano, salt, pepper, red wine vinegar, and extra virgin olive oil in a small bowl. Mix with a whisk.
4. Gently mix the salad with the dressing after drizzling it over it.
5. Serve right now for a tasty and refreshing salad alternative.

Broccoli Cheddar Soup

Prep time: 10 minutes
Cook time: 25 minutes
Servings: 4

Ingredients:

- 2 tbsps butter
- 1 small onion, diced
- 2 cloves garlic, minced
- 3 cup of of chopped broccoli florets
- 3 cup ofs of vegetable or chicken broth
- 1 cup of of milk
- 1 cup of of shredded cheddar cheese
- Salt and pepper to taste
- Optional: Croutons or extra shredded cheddar cheese for garnish

Instructions:

1. Keep the butter melted in a big pot over medium heat. In a sauté pan, cook the chopped onion and minced garlic for about three or four minutes or until the onion is nearly mushy.
2. The second step is to add the chopped broccoli florets to the saucepan with the vegetable or chicken broth. Gently boil the ingredients for about 15 minutes or until the broccoli florets are soft.

3. Next, thoroughly puree the soup using a blender or an immersion blender until it's completely smooth.
4. Put the soup back into the pot if it needs to be. As soon as the flour is incorporated, add the milk and shredded cheddar cheese. Continue stirring without interruption until the cheese melts and the soup becomes smooth and creamy.
5. Use salt and pepper according to your preference.
6. Top each bowl of soup with some shredded cheddar cheese, croutons, and the soup, if you want.
7. Enjoy the hearty soup with its reassuring broccoli and cheddar flavors when it's hot.

Mediterranean Chickpea Salad

Prep time: 15 minutes
Cook time: 0 minutes
Servings: 4

Ingredients:
- 2 cup ofs of cooked chickpeas
- 1 cucumber, diced
- 1 cup of of cherry tomatoes, halved
- Half a red onion, minced
- A quarter cup of of Kalamata olives, pitted and sliced
- 1/4 cup of of crumbled feta cheese
- 2 tbsps chopped fresh parsley
- 2 tbsps extra virgin olive oil
- 1 tbsp red wine vinegar
- Salt and pepper to taste

Instructions:
1. In a big basin, mix together the chickpeas, cucumber, cherry tomatoes, red onion, olives, feta cheese, and parsley.
2. A little bowl containing olive oil and red wine vinegar has to be whisked together to make the dressing. Salt and pepper to taste are the seasonings to use.
3. Toss the salad gently to coat all of the ingredients with the dressing.
4. Garnish with a garnish and serve right away or leave in the fridge until needed. Savour this fresh chickpea salad with a Mediterranean twist!

Chicken Noodle Soup

Prep time: 10 minutes
Cook time: 25 minutes
Servings: 6

Ingredients:
- 1 tbsp olive oil
- 1 onion, diced
- 2 carrots, sliced
- 2 celery stalks, sliced
- 2 cloves garlic, minced
- 6 cup ofs of chicken broth
- 2 cup ofs of cooked chicken breast, shredded

- 2 cup ofs of egg noodles
- 1 tsp dried thyme

- Salt and pepper to taste
- Optional: chopped fresh parsley

Instructions:

1. Melt the olive oil in a big saucepan over medium heat. Chopped carrots, celery, and onion should be added. The veggies should be softened after around 5 minutes of sautéing.
2. Once the minced garlic begins to smell, add it and continue cooking for another minute or two.
1. Bring the chicken broth to a boil after pouring it in.
3. Egg noodles, shredded chicken breast, and dried thyme should be stirred in before being brought to a boil. Make sure the noodles are tender before simmering for 10 to 12 minutes after boiling.
4. Make your own seasoning blend using salt and pepper.
5. Spoon the soup into individual dishes and, if preferred, top with freshly chopped parsley. Warm up some chicken noodle soup and savor it.

Caesar Salad with Homemade Croutons

Prep time: 15 minutes
Cook time: 10 minutes
Servings: 4

Ingredients:

- Wash and cut one head of romaine lettuce.
- 1 cup of of homemade croutons (see recipe below)

- ½ cup of of grated Parmesan cheese
- Caesar dressing (store-bought or homemade)

Instructions:

1. Chopped romaine lettuce and Caesar dressing should be mixed together in a big salad dish. Mix the lettuce until it's covered evenly.
2. Finish the salad by topping it with grated Parmesan.
3. Top with the homemade croutons.
4. Top with grilled chicken for a whole dinner, or serve right now as a side.

Minestrone Soup with Italian Sausage

Prep time: 15 minutes
Cook time: 30 minutes
Servings: 6

Ingredients:

- 1 tbsp olive oil
- 1 lb Italian sausage, casings removed
- 1 onion, diced

- 2 carrots, diced
- 2 stalks celery, diced
- 3 cloves garlic, minced
- 1 can (14.5 oz) diced tomatoes

- 6 cup ofs of chicken broth
- kidney beans, 15 ozs (one can), washed and drained
- 1 cup of of short pasta (like macaroni or ditalini)
- 2 tsp Italian seasoning
- Salt and pepper to taste
- Grated Parmesan cheese for serving

Instructions:

1. Melt the olive oil in a big saucepan over medium heat. While browning, crumble the Italian sausage with a spoon into tiny pieces.
2. Throw some chopped veggies (onion, carrots, celery, and garlic) into the saucepan. Once the veggies begin to soften, cook for another five to seven minutes.
3. Add the kidney beans, pasta, diced tomatoes, chicken broth, and Italian spice. Stir to combine. Reduce heat to low and simmer soup.
4. After around fifteen to 20 minutes of cooking, the pasta should be soft, and the flavors should be combined.
5. Make your own seasoning blend using salt and pepper.
6. If wanted, serve hot with grated Parmesan cheese as a garnish.

Asian Cucumber Salad with Sesame Ginger Dressing

Prep time: 15 minutes
Cook time: 0 minutes
Servings: 4

Ingredients:

- 2 cucumbers, thinly sliced
- 2 tbsps sesame oil
- 1 tbsp rice vinegar
- 1 tbsp soy sauce
- 1 tbsp honey
- 1 tsp freshly grated ginger
- 1 clove garlic, minced
- 1 tbsp sesame seeds
- Salt and pepper to taste
- 2 green onions, thinly sliced
- Optional: red pepper flakes for heat

Instructions:

1. In a small bowl, combine the sesame oil, rice vinegar, soy sauce, honey, garlic, ginger, sesame seeds, salt, and pepper. Whisk to combine.
2. Toss the green onions and sliced cucumbers in a big basin.
1. Toss the cucumber combination with the dressing until it is well covered.
3. If you like it hotter, add more red pepper flakes.
4. Enjoy right now, or keep it in the fridge until you're ready to dig in. Have fun!

Potato Leek Soup

Prep time: 10 minutes
Cook time: 30 minutes
Servings: 4

Ingredients

- 2-slice leeks, removing just the white and light green portions.
- 2 tbsps butter or olive oil
- 4 medium potatoes, peeled and diced
- 4 cup ofs of vegetable or chicken broth
- 1 cup of of milk or heavy cream
- Salt and pepper to taste
- Chopped chives or parsley for garnish (optional)

Instructions:

1. Heat the olive oil or butter over medium heat in a big saucepan.
2. Cook the sliced leeks for about 5 minutes or until they are tender.
3. Add the broth and potato cubes. The potatoes should be tender after 15–20 minutes of simmering covered.
4. Blend the soup until it's completely smooth using an immersion blender. Another option is to puree the soup in a blender before adding it back to the saucepan.
5. After seasoning with salt and pepper, stir in the milk or cream. Combine by stirring.
6. Cook, covered, for 5 to 10 more minutes or until well cooked.
1. Serve immediately, topping with chopped parsley or chives if preferred. Have fun!

Caprese Salad with Fresh Mozzarella and Basil

Prep time: 10 minutes
Cook time: 0 minutes
Servings: 4

Ingredients:

- 2 large ripe tomatoes, sliced
- 8 oz fresh mozzarella cheese, sliced
- 1/4 cup of of fresh basil leaves
- 2 tbsps extra virgin olive oil
- 2 tbsps balsamic glaze
- Salt and pepper to taste

Instructions:

1. On a serving dish, alternate the slices of tomato and mozzarella.
2. Step 2: Intersperse the tomato and mozzarella slices with fresh basil leaves.
3. The next step is to dress the salad with balsamic glaze and olive oil.
4. Spice it up with salt and pepper to taste.
5. Enjoy right away after serving!

Lentil Soup with Spinach and Lemon

Prep time: 10 minutes
Cook time: 30 minutes
Servings: 6

Ingredients:

- 1 tbsp olive oil
- 1 onion, chopped
- 2 carrots, diced
- 2 celery stalks, diced
- 2 cloves garlic, minced

- 1 cup of of dried green lentils,
  rinsed and drained
- 6 cup ofs of vegetable broth
- 2 cup ofs of fresh spinach leaves
- Juice of 1 lemon
- Salt and pepper to taste

Instructions:

1. A large saucepan set over medium heat should be used to warm the olive oil. Mix in the diced onion, celery, and carrots. For the vegetables, sauté for around 5 minutes or until they start to soften.
2. Cook the minced garlic for one more minute or until it begins to release its aroma.
3. Rinse the lentils and then throw them into the veggie stock. A boil is necessary, followed by a 20–25 minute simmer, to cook the lentils until they are soft.
4. Before serving, garnish the soup with fresh spinach leaves and squeeze in a little lemon juice. Stir occasionally and continue cooking for another 5 minutes or until the spinach has wilted.
5. Flavor with salt and pepper to taste.
6. Make this hearty lentil soup and serve it hot.

Waldorf Salad with Grilled Chicken

Prep time: 20 minutes
Cook time: 10 minutes
Servings: 4

Ingredients:

- 2 boneless, skinless chicken breasts
- Salt and pepper to taste
- 4 cup ofs of mixed salad greens
- 1 red apple, cored and diced
- 1 cup of of seedless grapes, halved
- 1/2 cup of of chopped celery
- 1/4 cup of of chopped walnuts
- 1/4 cup of of mayonnaise
- 2 tbsps Greek yogurt
- 1 tbsp lemon juice
- 1 tbsp honey
- 1 tsp Dijon mustard

Instructions:

1. Bring the grill up to a medium-high temperature.
2. Pepper and salt the chicken breasts.
3. Cook the chicken for four to five minutes on each side or until done. Let it sit for 5 minutes after taking it from the grill, and then slice it.
4. Toss together the salad greens, walnuts, celery, chopped apples, and grapes in a large basin.
5. To prepare the dressing, combine the mayonnaise, Greek yogurt, honey, lemon juice, and Dijon mustard in a small bowl and whisk to combine.
6. Sixth, top the salad with grilled chicken slices.
7. Evenly cover the salad with the dressing by drizzling dressing and tossing.
8. Take a bite and savor it!

Creamy Mushroom Soup

Prep time: 10 minutes
Cook time: 25 minutes
Servings: 4

Ingredients:

- 2 tbsps butter
- 1 onion, chopped
- 2 cloves garlic, minced
- 8 oz mushrooms, sliced
- 2 tbsps all-purpose flour
- 4 cup ofs of chicken or vegetable broth
- 1 cup of of heavy cream
- Salt and pepper to taste
- Chopped fresh parsley for garnish (optional)

Instructions:

1. Turn on a medium heat burner in a big pot and melt the butter.
2. Saute the chopped garlic and onion for three to four minutes or until they are tender.
3. Sauté the sliced mushrooms for 5 to 6 minutes or until they brown and lose their moisture.
4. Toss the mushrooms with the flour until they are uniformly coated. Add another two minutes of cooking time.
5. Add the broth, whether it's chicken or vegetable, slowly while stirring continuously to prevent lumps.
6. Reduce heat to medium and boil soup for 10–15 minutes or until slightly thickened.
7. Simmer for a further 5 minutes after stirring in the heavy cream.
8. Add salt and pepper according to your preference.
9. Spoon the soup into individual dishes and, if preferred, top with freshly chopped parsley.
10. Enjoy the luscious sweetness while it's hot!

Cobb Salad with Avocado and Bacon

Prep time: 15 minutes
Cook time: 15 minutes
Servings: 4

Ingredients:

- 8 cup ofs of mixed salad greens
- 2 cup ofs of cooked chicken breast, diced
- 4 hard-boiled eggs, sliced
- 1 cup of of cherry tomatoes, halved
- 1 cup of of cooked bacon, crumbled
- 1 avocado, diced
- 1/2 cup of of crumbled blue cheese

- 1/4 cup of of chopped red onion
- 1/4 cup of of chopped fresh parsley
- Salt and pepper to taste

Instructions:

1. Add the mixed salad greens, hard-boiled eggs, cherry tomatoes, crumbled bacon, avocado, blue cheese, red onion, and fresh parsley to a large salad bowl. Toss to combine.
2. Softly mix all of the salad ingredients by tossing the salad.
3. Add salt and pepper right before serving.
4. Get those plates ready and dig in!

Mexican Tortilla Soup

Prep time: 10 minutes
Cook time: 25 minutes
Servings: 6

Ingredients:

- 1 tbsp olive oil
- 1 onion, chopped
- 2 cloves garlic, minced
- 1 jalapeño pepper, seeded and chopped
- 1 tsp ground cumin
- 1 tsp chili powder
- 1/2 tsp dried oregano
- 6 cup ofs of chicken broth
- 1 can (14.5 oz) diced tomatoes
- 1 cup of of black bean sauce
- 1 cup of cooked black beans
- 1/4 cup of of chopped fresh cilantro
- Salt and pepper to taste
- Tortilla chips for serving
- Lime wedges for serving
- Avocado slices for serving
- Sour cream for serving

Instructions:

1. Melt the olive oil in a big saucepan over medium heat. Include the minced garlic, chopped jalapeño pepper, and chopped onion. Just give the onion a few minutes to soften in the pan.
2. Add the dried oregano, chili powder, and ground cumin. Stir to combine. Stir occasionally for another minute or two or until fragrant.
3. Add the chicken broth and tomato juices/chopped tomatoes. Simmer the soup for a few minutes.
4. Throw in the cooked black beans and corn kernels. To make sure all the flavors combine, simmer for about ten to fifteen minutes.
5. Incorporate the minced cilantro just before serving. When you're ready to season the soup, toss in some salt and pepper.
6. Serve the soup in individual bowls. Arrange the toppings: tortilla chips, avocado slices, lime wedges, and sour cream.

Spinach Strawberry Salad with Poppyseed Dressing

Prep time: 10 minutes

Cook time: 0 minutes
Servings: 4

Ingredients:

- 6 cup ofs of fresh baby spinach leaves
- 2 cup ofs of sliced strawberries
- 1/4 cup of of sliced almonds
- 1/4 cup of of crumbled feta cheese
- Red onion, thinly sliced, 1/4 cup of
- Slicing thinly one-quarter cup of of red onion

Instructions:

1. In a big basin, mix together the baby spinach leaves, sliced strawberries, sliced almonds, crumbled feta cheese, and thinly sliced red onion.
2. Top the salad with the poppyseed dressing.
3. Toss the salad ingredients gently to coat them with the dressing.
4. Get those plates ready and dig in!

Thai Coconut Curry Soup

Prep time: 10 minutes
Cook time: 20 minutes
Servings: 4

Ingredients:

- 1 tbsp coconut oil
- 1 onion, diced
- 2 cloves garlic, minced
- 1 tbsp grated ginger
- 2 tbsps Thai red curry paste
- 4 cup ofs of vegetable broth
- 1 can (14 oz) coconut milk
- Two cup ofs of chopped vegetables, such as bell peppers, zucchini, and carrots, are required by the recipe.
- 1 cup of of cooked chicken or tofu (optional)
- 2 tbsps soy sauce or tamari
- 1 tbsp lime juice
- Salt and pepper, to taste
- Fresh cilantro for garnish
- Cooked rice or noodles for serving (optional)

Instructions:

1. Cook the coconut oil in a large saucepan on medium heat until it fully melts. After the first five minutes, add the diced onion and continue sautéing until it starts to soften.Continue cooking for another minute or two or until the ginger and minced garlic begin to release their aroma.
2. After one more minute of cooking, stir in the Thai red curry paste.
3. Turn the heat down to a simmer and stir in the vegetable broth and coconut milk.
4. Toss in the chopped veggies and, if using, the cooked chicken or tofu. To make sure the veggies are soft, simmer for about ten to fifteen minutes.
5. Add the lime juice, salt, pepper, soy sauce (or tamari), and stir to combine.
6. Review the seasoning and make any necessary adjustments.

7. Hot soup with a sprinkle of fresh cilantro is ready to be served. It can be eaten on its own or topped with cooked rice or noodles.

CHAPTER 8:VEGETARIAN AND VEGAN OPTIONS

Quinoa Stuffed Bell Peppers

Prep time: 20 minutes
Cook time: 30 minutes
Servings: 4

Ingredients:

- 4 large bell peppers, any color
- 1 cup of of quinoa, rinsed
- 2 cup ofs of vegetable broth
- 1 tbsp olive oil
- 1 onion, diced
- 2 cloves garlic, minced
- 15 ozs (one can) of rinsed and drained black beans
- 1 cup of kernels of corn, fresh, frozen, or canned
- ground cumin, measuring 1 teaspoon
- 1 tsp chili powder
- Salt and pepper to taste
- 1 cup of of shredded cheese (optional)
- Fresh cilantro, chopped, for garnish

Instructions:

1. Heat oven to 190 degrees Celsius (375 degrees Fahrenheit). Before setting aside, coat a baking dish with olive oil.
2. Pluck the seeds and membranes from the bell peppers after removing the tops. Stand the bell peppers upright in the baking dish that you've prepared.
3. After you add the vegetable broth to the quinoa, stir it in a medium-sized saucepan. The quinoa needs fifteen to twenty minutes to boil, then simmer, covered, to cook and soak up the liquid.
4. Turn the olive oil to medium heat in a big skillet. 4. Chop some garlic and sauté some onion until it becomes translucent.
5. Combine cooked quinoa, black beans, corn, cumin, chili powder, salt, and pepper. After 5 more minutes of cooking, stir occasionally.
6. Toss the bell peppers with the quinoa mixture and distribute it evenly. As an option, you can sprinkle shredded cheese on top of every filled pepper.
7. Cook until the oven reaches 375 degrees Fahrenheit. For 25 to 30 minutes, or until the peppers are tender, bake them uncovered.
8. After taking it out of the oven, top it with chopped cilantro and serve. Have fun!

Vegan Lentil Shepherd's Pie

Prep time: 20 minutes
Cook time: 40 minutes
Servings: 6

Ingredients:

- 2 tbsps olive oil
- 1 onion, diced
- 2 carrots, diced
- 2 celery stalks, diced
- 3 cloves garlic, minced
- 1 cup of of dried green lentils, rinsed
- 3 cup ofs of vegetable broth
- 2 tbsps tomato paste
- 1 tsp dried thyme
- 1 tsp dried rosemary
- Salt and pepper to taste
- 4 cup ofs of mashed potatoes (homemade or store-bought)

Instructions:

1. Bring the oven temperature up to 375°F, which is 190°C. Before you put it aside, coat a 9-by-13-inch baking dish with olive oil.
2. Melt the olive oil in a big pan over medium heat. Chop some carrots, celery, and onion and throw them in. Just a few minutes in the sauté pan should be enough to soften the veggies.
3. Next, add the rinsed lentils, then the tomato paste, dried thyme, and rosemary, and finally the vegetable broth. Add salt and pepper to taste. Simmer, covered, for 25 to 30 minutes after boiling or until lentils are soft and liquid is absorbed.
1. Spread the lentil mixture evenly in the baking dish that you prepared in step four.
4. On top of the lentils, combine the mashed potatoes.
5. Preheat the oven to a preheated temperature and bake the mashed potatoes for 20-25 minutes or until they begin to lighten in color.
6. After taking it out of the oven, let it a few minutes to cool down before you dig in. Vegan Shepherd's Pie with Lentils—Enjoy

Eggplant Parmesan Bake

Prep time: 20 minutes
Cook time: 45 minutes
Servings: 4

Ingredients:

- Roughly chop one big eggplant into quarter-inch rounds.
- 2 cup of of marinara sauce
- 1 cup of of shredded mozzarella cheese
- 1/2 cup of of grated Parmesan cheese
- 1/2 cup of of breadcrumbs
- 2 tbsps olive oil
- 2 cloves garlic, minced
- Salt and pepper to taste

- Fresh basil leaves for garnish

Instructions:

1. Bring the oven temperature up to 375°F, which is 190°C. Apply olive oil to a baking dish.
2. In a colander, sprinkle some salt over the eggplant slices and leave them aside. Wait around 15 minutes for the excess water to evaporate. Roll up the slices in paper towels to dry them.
3. Combine the breadcrumbs, Parmesan cheese, garlic, salt, and pepper in a small bowl.
4. Evenly distribute half of the eggplant slices on the baking dish you just made. Toss half of the marinara sauce with the eggplant pieces before adding them.
5. Top the marinara sauce with half of the mozzarella cheese. Use the leftover eggplant, marinara sauce, and mozzarella cheese to stack the dish again.
6. Sprinkle the breadcrumb mixture over the dish.
7. Drizzle some olive oil on top to finish.
8. Place the baking dish, covered with foil, in the oven that has been prepared. After 30 minutes in the oven,
9. Bake, uncovered, for 15 more minutes or until cheese is melted and beginning to color. 9.
10. Let the dish rest for a few minutes before cutting and serving. Toss in some fresh basil leaves for garnish, if you want.

Spinach and Mushroom Risotto

Prep time: 10 minutes
Cook time: 30 minutes
Servings: 4

Ingredients:

- 1 cup of of Arborio rice
- 4 cup ofs of vegetable or chicken broth
- 1 onion, finely chopped
- 2 cloves garlic, minced
- 8 oz mushrooms, sliced
- 2 cup ofs of fresh spinach leaves
- 1/2 cup of of grated Parmesan cheese
- 2 tbsps butter
- 2 tbsps olive oil
- Salt and pepper to taste

- Fresh parsley for garnish (optional)

Instructions:

1. Bring the chicken or vegetable broth to a simmer in a saucepan. Maintain a warm temperature while you make the risotto.
2. The first step is to get the olive oil hot in a big skillet over medium heat. Once boiling, reduce heat and simmer for three or four more minutes, or until the chopped onion becomes translucent.
3. Cook for a further minute or two after adding the minced garlic or until a pleasant aroma begins to emanate.
4. Cook, covered, for 5 to 6 minutes or until the mushrooms soften and lose their liquid.
5. Add the Arborio rice and simmer, stirring occasionally, for one to two minutes or until golden brown.
6. Gradually add the heated broth to the pan, stirring without fail as you add each ladleful. Be careful not to add additional broth until the last one has been absorbed. About 20 to 25 minutes later, when the rice is cooked al dente and creamy, remove from the heat.
7. After approximately two or three minutes of cooking, add the fresh spinach leaves and toss to wilt.
8. Stop cooking the skillet and mix in the butter and grated Parmesan cheese until the butter melts and everything is mixed.
9. Add salt and pepper, seasoning to taste.
10. Hot risotto, topped with fresh parsley if preferred, is ready to be served.

Chickpea Tikka Masala

Prep time: 15 minutes
Cook time: 25 minutes
Servings: 4

Ingredients:

- Chickpeas, washed and drained, two cans (15 oz each
- 1 onion, diced
- 3 cloves garlic, minced
- 1 tbsp ginger, minced
- 1 bell pepper, diced
- 1 cup of of tomato sauce
- 1 cup of of coconut milk
- 2 tbsps tikka masala paste
- 1 tsp ground cumin
- 1 tsp ground coriander
- 1/2 tsp turmeric
- Salt and pepper to taste
- Fresh cilantro for garnish
- Cooked rice or naan bread for serving

Instructions:

1. One, in a big frying pan, heat the oil over medium heat. Incorporate finely chopped onion, garlic, and ginger. After around three to four minutes of sautéing, the onions should become transparent.

2. Cook for another two or three minutes after adding the diced bell pepper to the skillet.
3. Add turmeric, ground coriander, ground cumin, and tikka masala paste. Mix well. Toss for 30 seconds or until aromatic.
4. Mix in the coconut milk and tomato sauce by whisking well.
5. The chickpeas should be simmered for around 15–20 minutes or until the sauce becomes thick and the flavors combine.
6. Adjust with salt and pepper to taste. For garnish, sprinkle on some chopped cilantro.
7. Hot, served with cooked rice or naan bread, is step seven.

Vegan Chili with Cornbread Topping:

Prep time: 20 minutes
Cook time: 45 minutes
Servings: 6

Ingredients:
- 1 tbsp olive oil
- 1 onion, diced
- 2 cloves garlic, minced
- 1 bell pepper, diced
- 1 zucchini, diced
- 15 ozs (one can) of rinsed and drained black beans
- Kidney beans, drained and washed, one can (15 oz.)
- 1 can (15 oz) diced tomatoes
- 1 cup of of corn kernels, either fresh or frozen
- 2 tbsps chili powder
- 1 tsp ground cumin
- 1 tsp paprika
- Salt and pepper to taste
- 1 batch of prepared cornbread batter (use your favorite vegan recipe)

Instructions:
1. Bring the oven temperature up to 375°F, which is less than 190°C. Apply cooking spray to a baking dish that measures 9 by 13 inches.
2. Spread out the olive oil and heat it in a big pan over medium heat. Sauté the chopped onion and minced garlic for three or four minutes once they have gently softened.
3. Cook for another two or three minutes after adding diced zucchini and bell pepper to the pan. 4.
4. Combine the black beans, kidney beans, corn kernels, chopped tomatoes, chili powder, ground cumin, and paprika. Toss with salt and pepper according to taste. The flavors will combine after cooking for 10 to 15 minutes.
5. Evenly distribute the chili mixture into the baking dish that has been preheated.
6. Spread the cornmeal batter that has been made evenly over the chili mixture.
7. Cook the cornbread in a preheated oven for 25-30 minutes, or until it becomes a golden brown color and is fully done.
8. Get it out of the oven and give it a little time to cool down before you dig in.
9. Top with vegan sour cream, avocado, chopped green onions, or whatever else you choose while serving hot.

Butternut Squash and Sage Pasta

Prep time: 15 minutes
Cook time: 25 minutes
Servings: 4

Ingredients:

- Peel, seed, and cube one medium butternut squash.
- 8 oz whole wheat pasta
- 2 tbsps olive oil
- 2 cloves garlic, minced
- 1 tbsp fresh sage, chopped
- Salt and pepper to taste
- Grated Parmesan cheese (optional for serving)

Instructions:

1. Cook pasta according to package instructions. Drain and set aside.
2. Melt the olive oil in a big pan over medium-high heat. Add minced garlic and sauté until fragrant, about 1 minute.
3. Add cubed butternut squash to the skillet. Cook until squash is tender, stirring occasionally, about 15-20 minutes.
4. Stir in chopped sage and cooked pasta. Season with salt and pepper to taste.
5. Serve hot, optionally topped with grated Parmesan cheese.

Vegan Cauliflower Curry

Prep time: 15 minutes
Cook time: 30 minutes
Servings: 4

Ingredients:

- 1 medium head cauliflower, cut into florets
- 1 tbsp coconut oil
- 1 onion, diced
- 3 cloves garlic, minced
- 1 tbsp curry powder
- 1 tsp ground turmeric
- 1 can (14 oz) coconut milk
- 1 can (14 oz) diced tomatoes
- Salt and pepper to taste

- Fresh cilantro for garnish (optional)

Instructions:

1. In a large skillet or pan set over medium heat, melt the coconut oil. Add chopped onion and minced garlic. For the onions to get translucent, sauté them for around 5 minutes.
2. Chop some cauliflower and throw the florets into the pan. Slightly soften by cooking for about 5 minutes.
3. Coat the cauliflower evenly with the curry powder and turmeric.
4. The fourth step is to add the diced tomatoes, coconut milk, and tomato juices. Simmer, covered, for 15–20 minutes, or until curry thickens and cauliflower is soft.
5. Add pepper and salt to taste.
6. Top with chopped fresh cilantro and serve hot. Partake when dining on naan or rice.

Sweet Potato Black Bean Enchiladas

Prep time: 20 minutes
Cook time: 30 minutes
Servings: 6

Ingredients:

- 2 large sweet potatoes, peeled and diced
- 15 ozs (one can) of rinsed and drained black beans
- One sliced red bell pepper
- 1 onion, diced
- 2 cloves garlic, minced
- 1 tsp ground cumin
- 1 tsp chili powder
- Salt and pepper to taste
- 1 can (15 oz) enchilada sauce
- 8-10 whole wheat tortillas
- Cheddar or a Mexican mix shredded cheese, measuring 1 cup of
- Fresh cilantro for garnish (optional)

Instructions:

1. Involves baking at a temperature of 190 degrees Celsius (375 degrees Fahrenheit).
2. A large skillet set over medium heat should be used to warm the olive oil. 1. Finely mince the onion and mince the garlic. The onions should become translucent after about 5 minutes of cooking in the skillet.
3. Stir in the sweet potatoes and bell peppers, cubed. 3. Ten to fifteen minutes is approximately the right amount of time to cook sweet potatoes until they are absolutely soft.
4. Include the black beans, chili powder, and ground cumin in step four. Toss with salt and pepper according to taste. Sauté for another five minutes.
5. Apply a thin layer of enchilada sauce to a baking dish.
6. Arrange the tortillas seam-side down in the baking dish after filling them with the sweet potato and black bean mixture.
7. Top the rolled tortillas with the leftover enchilada sauce. Finally, top with shredded cheese.

8. Tent with foil and bake for twenty minutes. To get the desired melting and bubbling cheese, bake without the cover for an additional 5 to 10 minutes.
9. Before serving, garnish with fresh cilantro if preferred. Savor when hot.

Zucchini Noodles with Pesto

Prep time: 15 minutes
Cook time: 0 minutes
Servings: 2

Ingredients:
- 2 medium zucchinis, spiralized
- 1/2 cup of of fresh basil leaves
- 1/4 cup of of pine nuts
- 2 cloves garlic
- 1/4 cup of of grated Parmesan (to be added if you're not making it vegan)
- a quarter cup of of EVOO (40% olive oil)
- Salt and pepper to taste
- Cherry tomatoes (optional, for garnish)

Instructions:
1. To begin, throw the basil leaves, pine nuts, garlic, and (if using) Parmesan cheese into a food processor.
2. Pulse the items until they are finely minced.
3. While processing, drizzling in the olive oil little by little will result in a paste. Toss with salt and pepper according to taste.
4. Toss the spiralized zucchini in a big basin with the pesto until well coated.
5. Immediately serve with cherry tomatoes on top, if preferred.

Vegan Thai Coconut Soup

Prep time: 10 minutes
Cook time: 20 minutes
Servings: 4

Ingredients:
- 1 tbsp coconut oil
- 1 onion, diced
- 2 cloves garlic, minced
- 1 red bell pepper, sliced
- 1 tbsp grated ginger
- 2 tbsps Thai red curry paste
- 4 cup ofs of vegetable broth
- 1 can (14 oz) coconut milk

- 1 tbsp soy sauce
- 1 tbsp maple syrup
- Juice of 1 lime
- Salt and pepper to taste
- Fresh cilantro for garnish
- Red chili flakes for garnish (optional)

Instructions:

1. First, in a large saucepan set over medium heat, melt the coconut oil.
2. Add red bell pepper and grated ginger and cook for another 2 minutes.
3. Stir in Thai red curry paste and cook for 1 minute.
4. Pour in vegetable broth and coconut milk. Bring to a simmer and let it cook for 10 minutes.
5. Stir in soy sauce, maple syrup, and lime juice. Season with salt and pepper to taste.
6. Serve hot, garnished with fresh cilantro and red chili flakes if desired.

Portobello Mushroom Burgers

Prep time: 10 minutes
Cook time: 10 minutes
Servings: 2

Ingredients:

- 2 large portobello mushroom caps
- 2 tbsps balsamic vinegar
- 2 tbsps olive oil
- 1 tsp dried oregano
- 1 tsp garlic powder
- Salt and pepper to taste
- Burger buns
- Lettuce, tomato, and onion slices for topping

Instructions:

1. Get a grill or pan ready by heating it up over medium-high heat.
2. With a medium-sized saucepan, whisk or shake together the balsamic vinegar, olive oil, dried oregano, garlic powder, salt, and pepper.
3. Coat the portobello mushroom caps on both sides with the marinade.
4. Grill the mushroom caps with the gills facing down. Saute for five minutes.
5. After 5 minutes, turn the mushrooms over and continue grilling until they are soft.
6. If you'd like, toast the buns for the burgers on the grill.
7. Grill the portobello mushrooms and place them on the bottom half of the bread to assemble the burgers. Place the top half of the bread on top, then garnish with slices of onion, lettuce, and tomato.
8. Enjoy when it's hot!
9.

Vegan Tofu Stir-Fry

Prep time: 15 minutes
Cook time: 15 minutes
Servings: 4

Ingredients:
- 1 block (14 oz) of pressed and drained extra-firm tofu
- 2 tbsps soy sauce
- 1 tbsp sesame oil
- 1 tbsp cornstarch
- 2 tbsps vegetable oil
- 1 bell pepper, thinly sliced
- 1 cup of of broccoli florets
- 1 carrot, julienned
- 2 cloves garlic, minced
- 1 tbsp grated ginger
- 2 green onions, sliced
- Cooked rice or noodles for serving

Instructions:
1. Cover the pressed tofu cubes well with soy sauce, sesame oil, and cornstarch.
2. Boil some vegetable oil in a big wok or pan over medium-high heat. Toss in the cubes of tofu and sear them for 5-7 minutes or until they become golden crisp. Take out the tofu from the pan and put it aside.
3. Fry the bell pepper, broccoli, and carrot in the same pan until they are tender-crisp, which should take approximately 3 to 4 minutes. If necessary, add further oil.
4. Put the grated ginger and minced garlic back into the pan and let it simmer for one more minute.
5. Put the cooked tofu and sliced green onions back in the pan and simmer, stirring occasionally, until done.
6. Top the tofu stir-fry with cooked noodles or rice and serve hot. Have fun!

Lentil Walnut Loaf with Mushroom Gravy

Prep time: 20 minutes
Cook time: 1 hour
Servings: 6

Ingredients:
- 1 cup of of cooked lentils
- 1 cup of of chopped walnuts
- 1 small onion, finely chopped
- 2 cloves garlic, minced
- 1 carrot, grated
- 1 stalk celery, finely chopped
- 1 tbsp tomato paste
- 1 tbsp soy sauce
- 1 tsp dried thyme
- 1 tsp dried oregano
- 1/2 tsp smoked paprika
- Salt and pepper to taste
- 1/2 cup of of breadcrumbs
- 1/4 cup of of vegetable broth

Mushroom gravy:
- 2 cup of of sliced mushrooms
- 2 tbsps vegan butter
- 2 tbsps all-purpose flour
- 1 cup of of vegetable broth
- Salt and pepper to taste

Instructions:
1. Get the oven to 375°F, which is 190°C. Before you put it aside, grease a loaf pan.

2. The cooked lentils, chopped walnuts, onion, garlic, carrot, celery, tomato paste, soy sauce, dried thyme, dried oregano, smoked paprika, salt, and pepper should all be mixed together in a big mixing bowl. Blend well.
3. Stir in the breadcrumbs and vegetable broth until well-mixed with the mixture.
4. Carefully pour the batter into the loaf pan that has been preheated and push down firmly.
5. Lightly brown the top and make sure the lentil walnut loaf is solid when touched; this should take 45 to 50 minutes after preheating the oven.
6. Make the mushroom gravy while the bread is in the oven. The vegan butter should be melted in a pan set over medium heat. Sauté the sliced mushrooms until they soften and expel any excess liquid.
7. Dredge the mushrooms in the flour and toss to coat them evenly. Tend to the mixture for one or two minutes.
8. Add the vegetable broth gently while stirring constantly. Keep heating until the gravy thickens. Adjust the spices to your taste.
1. Wait a few minutes for the lentil walnut loaf to cool before cutting it. 9.
9. Spoon mushroom gravy over pieces of lentil walnut loaf and serve. Have fun!

Vegan Spinach and Artichoke Dip

Prep time: 15 minutes
Cook time: 25 minutes
Servings: 6

Ingredients:

- Raw cashews, one cup of, soaked in water for at least four hours and preferably overnight before draining.
- 1 tbsp olive oil
- 1 small onion, finely chopped
- 2 cloves garlic, minced
- 1 (14-oz) can artichoke hearts, drained and chopped
- 2 cup ofs of fresh spinach, chopped
- 1 cup of of unsweetened almond milk
- 1/4 cup of of nutritional yeast
- 1 tbsp lemon juice
- 1 tsp garlic powder
- 1/2 tsp onion powder
- Salt and pepper to taste

Instructions:

1. Turn the oven on high heat (around 190°C, or 375°F). Spray or coat a baking dish with olive oil to prevent sticking.
2. Put the almond milk and soaked cashews into a blender or food processor. Mix till light and fluffy. Remove off the table.
3. To preheat the olive oil, place a skillet over medium heat. In a sauté pan, mince the garlic and onion. The veggies should be tender and aromatic after frying for three or four minutes.

4. Toss in the chopped spinach and artichoke hearts in the skillet. Swallow the spinach for two or three minutes or until it wilts.
5. Add the nutritional yeast, cashew-almond milk combination, lemon juice, onion and garlic powders, salt, and pepper, whisking until combined. Mix well by whisking. Heat through and mix, stirring periodically for another two to three minutes.
6. Evenly distribute the mixture into the baking dish that has been prepared.
7. The dip should be bubbling and somewhat golden in color after 20 to 25 minutes in a preheated oven.
8. Take it out of the oven and set it aside to cool for a while before cutting and serving. Dip it in your preferred condiment and serve with bread, crackers, or veggie sticks.

Mediterranean Quinoa Salad

Prep time: 15 minutes
Cook time: 15 minutes
Servings: 4

Ingredients:

- 1 cup of of quinoa, rinsed and drained
- 2 cup ofs of water or vegetable broth
- 1 cup of of cherry tomatoes, halved
- 1/2 English cucumber, diced
- Half a cup of of pitted Kalamata olives
- Red onion, finely chopped, 1/4 cup of
- a quarter cup of of chopped fresh parsley
- Chop 1/4 cup of of fresh mint.
- One-fourth cup of of extra-virgin olive oil
- 2 tbsps lemon juice
- 1 clove garlic, minced
- 1 tsp dried oregano
- Salt and pepper to taste
- Optional: crumbled feta cheese for garnish (omit if vegan)

Instructions:

1. Put the quinoa and some water or vegetable broth in a medium pot. On a high flame, bring to a boil.
2. Cover and simmer the quinoa for about 15 minutes over low heat to cook until it absorbs all the water. After five minutes of sitting covered, take it out of the oven. Once cooled to room temperature, toss the quinoa in a bowl using a fork.
3. In a big basin, mix together the cooked quinoa, cucumber, olives, cherry tomatoes, red onion, parsley, and mint.
4. To create the dressing, pour olive oil into a small bowl and whisk in the lemon juice, chopped garlic, dried oregano, salt, and pepper.
5. Toss the quinoa salad with the dressing until it coats all of the ingredients.
6. Before serving, taste the spice and adjust as needed. You may top the salad with crumbled feta cheese if you choose.

7. Right now or store in the fridge for later. 7. You may have this salad as a light lunch or serve it as a side dish with grilled chicken, veggies, or fish.

Vegan Black Bean Tacos with Mango Salsa

Prep time: 15 minutes
Cook time: 15 minutes
Servings: 4

Ingredients:

- 15 ozs of black beans, washed and drained–1 can
- One sliced ripe mango
- 1 small red onion, finely chopped
- 1 jalapeño pepper, seeded and minced
- 1/4 cup of of fresh cilantro, chopped
- Juice of 1 lime
- Salt to taste
- 8 small corn tortillas
- Optional toppings: avocado slices, shredded lettuce, hot sauce

Instructions:

1. Mix together the black beans, mango, red onion, cilantro, and minced jalapeño pepper in a medium bowl.
2. Toss the ingredients lightly to blend after adding the lime juice. Taste and add salt as desired.
3. Make sure the corn tortillas are soft and malleable by warming them in a pan over medium heat.
1. Transfer the black bean mixture to each tortilla using a spoon.
4. Top the tacos with shredded lettuce, avocado slices, and spicy sauce if desired.
5. Vegan black bean tacos topped with mango salsa are ready to be enjoyed!

Spaghetti Squash Pad Thai

Prep time: 10 minutes
Cook time: 25 minutes
Servings: 2

Ingredients:

- 1 medium spaghetti squash
- 2 tbsps olive oil

- 2 cloves garlic, minced
- 1 red bell pepper, thinly sliced
- 1 carrot, julienned
- 2 green onions, chopped
- 1/4 cup of of peanuts, chopped
- 2 tbsps soy sauce or tamari
- 1 tbsp maple syrup or agave nectar
- 1 tbsp rice vinegar
- Juice of 1 lime
- Sriracha sauce (optional)
- Fresh cilantro for garnish

Instructions:

1. Get the oven to 400°F or 200°C. Separate the spaghetti squash's seeds and cut it lengthwise in half.
2. On a parchment-lined baking sheet, lay the squash pieces cut side down. To make sure the squash is soft and readily punctured, bake it for 25-30 minutes. Allow to cool for a little while.
3. Lightly coat a big pan with olive oil and set it over medium heat while the squash bakes. One minute before the garlic becomes aromatic, add the minced garlic.
4. Toss into the pan some sliced red bell pepper, julienned carrot, and chopped green onions. Simmer for 5 to 7 minutes or until the veggies are soft and slightly crunchy.
1. 5-Scrape the flesh of the spaghetti squash into strands with a fork. Cook the veggies in a pan and then add the strands of squash.
5. Whisk together the lime juice, rice vinegar, soy sauce, maple syrup, and maple syrup in a small basin. Toss the squash and vegetables in the pan with the sauce. Mix everything together to coat.
6. To ensure complete heating, continue cooking for another two to three minutes. 7.
7. Garnish each serving of Spaghetti Squash Pad Thai with chopped peanuts, fresh cilantro, and sriracha sauce, if preferred.
8. Slurp up the tasty Spaghetti Squash Pad Thai!

Vegan Chickpea Salad Sandwiches

Prep time: 15 minutes
Cook time: 0 minutes
Servings: 4 sandwiches

Ingredients:

- 1 can of washed and drained chickpeas (15 oz.)
- 1/4 cup of of vegan mayonnaise
- 1 tbsp Dijon mustard
- 2 tbsps finely chopped red onion
- 2 tbsps finely chopped celery
- 1/3 cup of fresh dill, chopped (or 1/4 teaspoon dried dill)
- 1 tbsp lemon juice
- Salt and pepper to taste
- 8 slices whole grain bread
- Lettuce leaves
- Sliced tomatoes
- Sliced cucumbers

Instructions:

1. Mash the chickpeas well in a medium-sized basin using a fork or potato masher, ensuring that they retain some pieces.

2. Mash the chickpeas and mix in vegan mayonnaise, Dijon mustard, red onion, celery, dill, lemon juice, salt, and pepper. Blend well by stirring.
3. If you'd like, toast the pieces of whole-grain bread.
4. Top four pieces of bread with the chickpea salad.
5. Garnish with sliced cucumbers, tomatoes, and lettuce leaves.
6. Put the other pieces of bread on top to create sandwiches.
7. Wrap firmly in plastic wrap or foil and serve right away, or package tightly for later pleasure.

Roasted Vegetable and Hummus Wraps

Prep time: 15 minutes
Cook time: 25 minutes
Servings: 4

Ingredients:

- twocup ofs of sliced mixed veggies (eggplant, bell peppers, zucchini, red onion, etc.)
- 1 tbsp olive oil
- Salt and pepper to taste
- 4 large whole wheat or spinach wraps
- 1 cup of of hummus
- Handful of baby spinach leaves
- Handful of alfalfa sprouts (optional)
- Sliced avocado (optional)

Instructions:

1. Set oven temperature to 400°F or 200°C.
2. Finish up the mixed vegetables by adding the olive oil, salt, and pepper. Put in the coat. Line a baking sheet with them.
3. Roast the veggies in a preheated oven for 20-25 minutes, stirring halfway through or until they are soft and slightly browned.
4. Preheat a dry skillet over medium heat for about 30 seconds on each side, or pop the wraps in the microwave for a few seconds.
5. Leave a border around the sides of each wrap and spread 1/4 cup of of hummus on top.
6. Before serving, top the hummus with roasted veggies, spinach, alfalfa sprouts, and sliced avocado, if desired.
7. After placing the filling in the center, fold the edges of the wrap over it. Starting from the bottom, roll it securely.
8. Serve right away after slicing the wraps diagonally in half, if preferred.

Chapter 9: Savory Beef And Pork Recipes

Tangy BBQ Pulled Pork

Prep time: 30 minutes
Cook time: 5 hours
Servings: 5

Ingredients:

- 1 boneless pork shoulder (around 6 ibslib)
- ¼ C dark brown sugar
- 1 tsp cayenne pepper
- 2 tsp cumin
- 1 Tbsp paprika
- 1 Tbsp chile powder
- 1 tsp cracked pepper
- 2 tsp kosher salt
- 1 Tbsp olive oil
- 3 yellow onions. quartered
- 2 large carrots, chopped into large pieces
- 6 cloves garlic
- 2 C chicken stock
- brioche buns or Hawaiian rolls
- Your favorite BBQ sauce or GTK BBQ sauce - see the recipe below

For the Homemade BBQ Sauce:

- 2 C ketchup
- ½ C brown sugar
- ⅓ C Worcestershire sauce
- ¼ C cider vinegar
- 1 Tbsp hot pepper sauce (we use smokey chipotle pepper sauce) -

adjust based on the amount of heat you prefer

- 4 cloves garlic - minced
- 2 tsp dry mustard powder
- 1 Tbsp liquid smoke
- ¼ C molasses
- 1 tsp kosher sa

For the Tangy Slaw:

- ½ head napa cabbage - thinly sliced
- ½ head purple cabbage - thinly sliced
- ¼ C cider vinegar
- ¼ C oil (we used peanut oil)
- 1 Tbsp honey
- ¼ tsp dry mustard
- ¼ tsp celery salt

Instructions:

In regards to the Barbecue Pork:

1. Make a small bowl and add brown sugar, cayenne pepper, cumin, paprika, chilli powder, salt, and pepper. Combine everything by blending it.
2. Rub the pork all over its outside. Place pork in the refrigerator, tightly wrapped in plastic, for at least four hours, or ideally all night.
3. Put in the oven and bake for three minutes at 325 degrees. In a heavy saucepan or Dutch oven set over medium-high heat, brown the pork for about 2 minutes on each side after adding the olive oil.
4. When the meat is well browned, cook the pork on top of the onions, carrots, and garlic that have been added to the pan's base. Put the chicken stock in the pan, cover it with the lid, and bake it.
5. The meat should be fork-tender and easily pulled apart after about five hours of cooking.
6. After removing from the oven, take the meat and onions to a chopping board. Chop the meat into big pieces and place in a basin.

7. Toss the meat to coat it with the BBQ sauce and pour it over to your liking.

Regarding the Homemade Barbecue Sauce:

1. First, combine everything in a medium bowl and whisk to combine

Regarding the Spicy Slaw:

1. Initial step: boil vinegar, oil, and honey in a small pot. Put the celery salt and dry mustard in after you take it off the heat. Stir the ingredients until well combined, then set aside to cool. Stir in the cooled cabbage and onion mixture. Add the mixture and whisk well to coat.
2. Make and chill the slaw in the fridge.

Classic Beef Stew

Prep time: 15 minutes
Cook time: 1 hour 30 minutes
Servings: 6

Ingredients:

- Ingredients: 2 lbs of cubed beef stew meat
- 1 ½ teaspoons kosher salt
- ½ teaspoon freshly ground black pepper
- 2 tbsps extra virgin olive oil
- 1 large yellow onion, cut into chunks
- 4 garlic cloves, minced
- 2 tbsps red wine vinegar
- 1 tbsp tomato paste
- 2 tbsps arrowroot powder, cornstarch, or other flour
- 1 cup of red wine
- 4 cups of low-sodium beef broth
- ½ teaspoon dried thyme
- 2 bay leaves
- 1 ibslib baby white potatoes, halved or quartered
- Use four medium carrots that have been peeled and cut diagonally.
- 3 celery ribs, chopped
- Optional: fresh thyme for garnish

Instructions:

1. Season the meat, don't forget. Pressing it with paper towels will help dry the meat. Toss with a pinch of salt and a squeeze of pepper.
2. A last sear will finish cooking the meat. A large stockpot or Dutch oven should be prepared over medium-high heat to heat the oil. Do not crowd the pan; brown the meat in batches, 2–3 minutes on each side. Move to a serving dish after the sear has finished.
3. A last sear will finish cooking the meat. A large stockpot or Dutch oven should be prepared over medium-high heat to heat the oil. Do not crowd the pan; brown the meat in batches, 2–3 minutes on each side. Move to a serving dish after the sear has finished.
4. Bring the meat back to a simmer. Return the steak to the saucepan after searing it, and sprinkle some flour on top. Once the flour is completely dissolved, stir in the other ingredients.

5. Pour in the aromatics and liquids. Pour in the broth, thyme, bay leaf, wine, and thyme. Incorporate all ingredients by use of a spatula or a big spoon. The soup should be brought to a boil, then simmered, partly covered, for an hour over low heat.
6. Put the vegetables in. Incorporate the celery, carrots, and potatoes. After the first 20 to 30 minutes, continue cooking until the veggies are soft to the touch.
7. Take a seat. Before serving, take out the bay leaves and, if desired, top with fresh thyme.

Spicy Beef Tacos

Prep time: 15 minutes
Cook time: 30 minutes
Servings: 4

Ingredients:

- 1 tbsp sunflower oil
- 1 onion chopped
- 1 red chilli seeded and chopped
- 2 cloves garlic crushed
- 500 g lean minced beef
- 4 ripe tomatoes chopped
- 300 g can red kidney beans rinsed and drained

- 2 tsp paprika
- 1 teaspoon hot chilli powder Optional
- 1 teaspoon ground cumin
- 1 teaspoon ground coriander
- 1 teaspoon oregano
- salt and freshly ground black pepper

To Serve:

- 12 taco shells
- guacamole

- spicy tomato salsa
- grated cheddar cheese

Instructions:

1. In a tablespoon of oil, sauté one chopped onion and one chopped chili for about 5 minutes, or until the onions and chilies are soft. Toss in two cloves of crushed garlic and stir to combine.
2. Meanwhile, the mince cooks split it up with a spoon, and add 500g (1 lb 2 oz). Brown it.
3. Add 2 teaspoons of paprika, 1 teaspoon of each chili powder (if using), cumin, coriander, and oregano, and mix well.
4. Sauté 4 chopped tomatoes and 4 drained cans of red kidney beans (400g, or 14 oz) for 30 minutes on low heat. According to your preference, add seasoning.

To serve:

1. Follow the package directions to heat the taco shells.
2. Spoon the meat filling into the shells and top with a little guacamole, salsa, and cheese. Serve immediately.

Garlic Herb Pork Chops

Prep time: 10 minutes
Cook time: 4 minutes
Servings: 4

Ingredients:
- 4 oz each of thinly sliced bone-in pork chops
- 1 tbsps extra virgin olive oil
- ¾ teaspoon crushed dried rosemary
- ½ teaspoon dried sage
- ½ teaspoon paprika
- ½ teaspoon salt
- ½ teaspoon ground pepper

The Butter:
- 4 teaspoons unsalted butter at room temperature
- 1 garlic clove minced
- ½ teaspoon crushed dried rosemary

Instructions:
1. Get a shallow dish or mixing bowl and lay the pork chops on top.
2. In a little bowl, combine the olive oil and ¾ teaspoon of rosemary, sage, paprika, salt, and pepper. Once the marinade is poured over the pork chops, massage them to spread the flavor.
3. Bring a large nonstick skillet to a medium-high temperature. Generously coat with nonstick cooking spray.
4. After three minutes on one side and one more minute on the other, or until cooked through, turn the pork chops over. Evenly distribute the pork chops among four plates. Spoon one teaspoon of garlic butter on top of each chop.

The Butter:
1. Get a small bowl and mix the butter, garlic, and rosemary together.

Beef and Broccoli Stir-Fry

Prep time: 10 minutes
Cook time: 20 minutes
Servings: 4

Ingredients:
- Thinly cut flank steak, 1 1/4 ibslib
- 1 tbsp + 1 teaspoon vegetable oil divided use
- 2 cup of broccoli florets
- 2 teaspoons minced fresh ginger
- 1 teaspoon minced garlic
- 1/4 cup of oyster sauce
- Beef broth (or water) measuring 1/4 cup
- 1 teaspoon sugar
- 2 teaspoons toasted sesame oil
- 1 teaspoon soy sauce
- 1 teaspoon cornstarch
- salt and pepper to taste

Instructions:
1. In a big skillet, heat up 1 teaspoon of oil over medium heat. Before the broccoli is cooked, add it to the pan and fry for about 4 minutes.
2. Sauté the garlic and ginger for another 30 seconds.
3. Take the broccoli out of the pan, transfer it to a platter, and then cover it.

4. Heat the pan over high heat after wiping it down with a paper towel. Pour in the other tbsp of oil.
5. If you're cooking in batches, season the steak with salt and pepper before adding it to the pan in a single layer. Once browned and cooked through, sauté for another 3 to 4 minutes each side.
6. Return the broccoli mixture to the skillet and reheat it for another two minutes or until it is no longer raw.
7. Blend the oyster sauce, sugar, sesame oil, soy sauce, beef broth, and sesame seeds in a mixing bowl. A spoonful of cold water and cornflour should be mixed in a small bowl.
8. After 30 seconds, stir in the meat and vegetables with the oyster sauce combination and return to the heat. Combine the cornflour with the sauce ingredients and cook for one more minute or until the sauce starts to thicken.
9. Quickly serve with rice on the side, if preferred.

Slow Cooker Pork Carnitas

Prep time: 5 minutes
Cook time: 7 hours
Servings: 10

Ingredients:
- 2 kilograms of pork shoulder, with excessive amounts of fat removed.
- One peeled and sliced onion
- Two limes, half-cut
- One half of an orange
- Two teaspoons of salt
- two teaspoons of ground cumin
- Two teaspoons of dried oregano
- Ground black pepper on a fresh basis

Instructions:
1. Add the onion and pork shoulder to the slow cooker.
2. Toss the pork with the squeezed lime and orange juices and garnish with the squeezed fruits.
3. Toss in the cumin, oregano, salt, and pepper. Season to taste.
4. Take the lid off and let it cook on HIGH for seven or eight more hours or on LOW for eleven or twelve more hours until it easily flakes with a fork.
5. After cooking, remove the meat from the cooking liquids (refrain from discarding them!) and chop it into bite-sized pieces. Top with a baking sheet that can withstand being placed on a grill.
6. Flip the meat over once or twice while it's under the grill for 5 to 10 minutes or until some of the "prickly" parts are browned and crispy.
7. Toss the fruit out of the cooking liquid and return the crispy pork to it, stirring to combine.

Savory Beef Shepherd's Pie

Prep time: 10 minutes
Cook time: 75 minutes
Servings: 8

Ingredients:

- 1 ½ – 2 Lbs. Ground Beef
- Half a cup of finely chopped onion
- 2 teaspoons of minced garlic
- Chopsticks (4 tablespoons)
- Ingredients: 1 package of frozen mixed vegetables (corn, carrots, and green beans).
- 2 Tbsps Flour (I use Bob Mills)
- 1 ½ Cup of Beef stock or broth
- 2 teaspoons Worcestershire sauce
- 4–6 oz cheese, freshly grated (I use cheddar)
- Mashed potatoes (Between 1 ½ – 2 lbs)

Instructions:

1. Prep the oven to 500 degrees Fahrenheit.
2. Before adding the onion, heat up the oil in a large pan. Cook, turning regularly, until the onion begins to become translucent, around four or five minutes. Mix in a pinch of pepper and a pinch of salt. Keeping the heat low helps prevent the onion from browning.
3. Toss in the garlic and mix it in with the onion for around a minute.
4. Put the meat back in the pan and add the salt and pepper. Once cooked, split up with a fork to prevent sticking. Should it be required, drain.
5. After 1 minute, sprinkle the flour evenly over the grill. Include the Spaghetti sauce, beef stock, and Worcestershire sauce. If you want a rich gravy, simmer it for 5–10 minutes on low heat.
6. Line a 913 casserole dish with the beef mixture, and then add the veggies in layers.
7. Toss with the crumbled cheese.
8. Evenly distribute the mashed potatoes over the top, being sure to cover all the meat and cheese.
9. Since the meat is fully cooked, browning the potatoes is the only remaining step. Gently place the casserole dish on the grill until the potatoes get a beautiful golden brown crust. This may need 5–10 minutes.

Honey Mustard Glazed Pork Tenderloin

Prep time: 20 minutes
Cook time: 40 minutes
Servings: 2

Ingredients:

- 2 teaspoons dried oregano
- 1 teaspoon dried parsley flakes
- 1/2 teaspoon dried rosemary, crushed
- 1/2 teaspoon dried thyme
- 1/2 teaspoon garlic powder
- 1/2 teaspoon seasoned salt
- Dash pepper
- Dash cayenne pepper
- 1 pork tenderloin (3/4 ibslib)

Glaze:

- 4-1/2 teaspoons brown sugar
- 4-1/2 teaspoons Dijon mustard
- 1/4 teaspoon honey

Instructions:

1. Take a small bowl and mix together the first eight ingredients. Put the rub on the meat. Seal and store in a big plastic bag. Place in the fridge for at least one night after processing.
2. The glaze components should be combined. Steep the tenderloin in a shallow roasting pan lined with foil. Cook, basting periodically with glaze, for 40–45 minutes uncovered at 350° or until a thermometer registers 160°. Before slicing, let it stand for 5 minutes.

Beef and Mushroom Risotto

Prep time: 15 minutes
Cook time: 1 hour 45 minutes
Servings: 8

Ingredients:

- 600g gravy beef, fat trimmed
- 2 brown onions
- 3 fresh thyme sprigs, plus 1 tbsp extra leaves
- 1 bay leaf
- 1 1/2 L (6 cups of) beef stock
- 2 tbsp olive oil
- 2 garlic cloves, crushed
- 400 g (2 cup ofs) arborio rice
- 125ml (1/2 cup of) dry white wine
- 1 bunch asparagus, cut into 2cm lengths
- 1/3 cup of (25gm) finely grated parmesan cheese, plus extra, to serve
- 60g baby spinach
- 400g mixed mushrooms, sliced
- Zest of 1 lemon
- Lemon wedges to serve
- Parsley leaves to serve
- Baby Rocket leaves to serve

Instructions:

1. One onion, peeled and minced. Put chopped onion, thyme, bay leaf, and boiled stock into a large saucepan. Then, add the animal. Add the cover and continue cooking for another hour over low heat until the meat is very soft.
2. Making use of a slotted spoon, Insert a slotted spoon into the cooking liquid and lift the meat out. Meat should be coarsely shredded. After heating, strain the liquid into a medium saucepan; throw away the sediments. Heat the stock mixture covered.
3. Dice the leftover onion finely. On medium heat, in a big saucepan, heat half of the oil. For 5 minutes, while stirring occasionally, soften the onion. Sauté the garlic for 1 minute while stirring occasionally. Mix in the rice and thyme leaves, then toss for a minute or two to coat.
4. Whisk in the wine at regular intervals to keep it from evaporating while you bring the mixture to a boil. Turn the heat down to low. Carefully add ladles of hot stock one at a time, whisking constantly, and let each one soak. Stir in the asparagus and keep cooking for a further 5 minutes after 25 to 30 minutes, or until the rice reaches an al dente texture and the liquid is absorbed. Put the Parmesan and spinach into the pan after taking it off the heat. Before serving, adjust the seasoning to taste. Set aside, covered, for two minutes.
5. Keep the remaining oil warm in a big nonstick skillet over medium-high heat. Once the mushrooms have softened, cook them for 5 minutes while stirring occasionally. Before stirring the risotto, add the steak and mushrooms.
6. Lemon wedges and young rocket leaves are served on the side, and the risotto is topped with parsley, lemon zest, and the remaining Parmesan.

Pork and Vegetable Skewers

Prep time: 20 minutes
Cook time: 10 minutes
Servings: 4

Ingredients:

- 2 tbsps extra virgin olive oil
- 2 teaspoons Dijon mustard
- 1 teaspoon paprika
- 1/2 teaspoon granulated garlic
- 1/2 teaspoon light brown sugar
- 1/2 teaspoon kosher salt
- 1/4 teaspoon fresh ground pepper
- 1 1/4 ibslib boneless pork sirloin, cut into 1-inch cubes
- 8 cherry tomatoes
- 1/2 small yellow squash, cut into 1/4 inch rounds
- 1/2 green zucchini, cut into 1/4 inch rounds

Instructions:

1. Stir the garlic paste, olive oil, mustard, and dry ingredients in a medium-sized bowl until combined. Toss the meat with the marinade and coat it evenly.
2. After 10–15 minutes, set aside to cool before grilling. Make sure to dip the skewers in water while the meat is marinating so they don't burn.

3. Heat grill.
4. Thread the pork and vegetables onto skewers, alternating ingredients. Any combination of vegetables can be used.
5. Grill over high heat until pork is barely pink, approximately 4-6 minutes.
6. Turn once during grilling.
7. Serve warm.

Beef Chilli Con Carne

Prep time: 2 minutes
Cook time: 120 minutes
Servings: 4

Ingredients:

- Fifty grams of high-quality minced beef or stewing steak
- Minced onions, two big
- Three hundred and fifty grams of delicious red pepper, like Florina, each. two not cut and one entire
- Minced garlic, three cloves
- tomato paste (2 tablespoons)
- 1–2 tablespoons of red wine vinegar
- a dark chocolate chunk or one tablespoon of date syrup
- 160–200 milliliters of chicken or beef stock. Maybe not everything on this list is necessary.
- 1.5 kilograms of red kidney beans, 400 grams of pinto beans, or both
- olive oil
- salt and freshly ground black pepper

Spices:

- 1 tsp cumin
- ½ tsp cinnamon
- small stick cinnamon
- ¼ tsp powdered allspice
- ¼ tsp powdered cloves
- 1 tsp dried oregano
- 1 bay leaf

Chillis:

- 4 small dried red chillies
- 1 large ancho or banana chili pepper I struggle to find ancho, so I have to substitute ancho for the local banana chili. You will need to soak the ancho chili.
- 2 chipotle in adobo sauce, incl. 2 tsp of the sauce
- Serving Suggestions
- 1 lime
- 1 handful fresh coriander
- 200 ml yogurt or sour cream
- beans, rice, tortillas, nachos, burritos, tacos…. or spaghetti
- Grated cheese if you are using spaghetti
- guacamole

Instructions:

1. Season the meat with black pepper and brown it on both sides in a separate skillet with a little amount of oil.
2. At the same time, roast the dried chilies (to release their taste) until they are fragrant, but not browned. After removing, place them in a small dish with a splash of boiling water and, if using, the ancho chilli. Permit to melt.
3. In a skillet or oven, roast two sweet red peppers. Remember, don't burn them; just soften them evenly and set them aside.
4. Sauté the onions and diced sweet red pepper in olive oil. While the onion is softening and becoming translucent, add all of the dry spices, along with the bay leaf and cinnamon stick.
5. In a little food processor, chopped sweet red pepper, sliced banana or ancho chilli, softened dried chilies, two tablespoons tomato paste, chipotle in adobo sauce, garlic, and a spoonful of cooked onions should be mixed in while the onions are cooking. The mixture should be pulsed until it becomes a thick paste. Just add a little stock to thin it down before you blend it.
6. After stirring for a few minutes, add the meat and the chili mixture to the onions. Cook, stirring occasionally.
7. Pour 1/4 cup of stock into the food processor and pulse until you have all the chili sauce; then pour it over the chili.
8. Once the chilli is boiling, add the date syrup and red wine vinegar. Slightly ajar cover and simmer on low heat until meat is cooked and sauce thickens. To maintain the moisture of the chilli, add ½ cup of stock gradually.
9. Instead of boiling it in a lot of water, simmer it slowly. Approximately one and a half to two hours is required.
10. The beans, if used, should be added 30 minutes into the cooking time.
11. Allow the meat to cool and refrigerate for at least one more night when it has reached a soft consistency.
12. Reheat gently before serving; add extra liquid if needed. Season to taste; add salt or vinegar if needed. Adjust the level of heat to your preference; this is a medium-hot pepper.
13. See the notes for the suggested accompaniments.

Apple Cider Braised Pork Shoulder

Prep time: 20 minutes
Cook time: 3 hours 45 minutes
Servings: 4

Ingredients:

- 4-5 pound roasts of pork, preferably Boston butt or pork shoulder
- 2 tbsps neutral oil
- 2 cups of fresh apple cider* (not apple cider vinegar)
- 2 cups of chicken stock or broth
- 2 tbsps dijon mustard
- 1 tbsp dehydrated minced onion

- 1 head of garlic, top sliced off opposite of the root end
- 3 rosemary sprigs
- 4 thyme sprigs
- 1 red onion, cut into thick slices
- 2 firm and slightly tart apples*, peeled and cut into wedges
- kosher salt
- freshly cracked black pepper

Instructions:

1. Warm up the oven to 325 degrees Fahrenheit.
2. If there are big globs of fat on the pork, remove them first. Pork, if bone-in, may be left whole or cut into four big pieces.
3. After patting the pork with a paper towel, generously sprinkle kosher salt and pepper over the whole piece.
4. The oil should be heated in a big Dutch oven over medium-high heat. Lay down one layer of pork and drop it into the hot oil. After four or five minutes of searing, the pork should be perfectly browned on both sides. Turn around and repeat the process. For smaller Dutch ovens, you may need to cook in batches.
5. Toss the cider, stock or broth, dijon mustard, and dehydrated chopped onion with the pork as it cooks on the grill. Gather some thyme and rosemary and bind them in a little bundle using kitchen twine.
6. Pour the braising liquid over the meat when it has browned evenly. Put the pork, garlic head, and herbs in a saucepan, cover, and bake for 30 minutes.
7. The pork should be braised for about three hours, turning it over halfway through. If using boneless pigs, begin checking after two and a half hours. Before arranging the pork with the apples and onions, take it out of the oven when it's almost fork-soft. Set the oven timer for 30–45 minutes more and cover it. By now, the pork ought to be very juicy.
8. After taking the pork out of the oven, let it aside to rest for 30 minutes in the braising liquid. Shuck the garlic cloves and either throw them into the stock or press them into the meat. Add salt and pepper to the braising liquid according to your taste. The pork, apples, and onions should be served with the juices spooned over them.

Beef and Spinach Lasagna

Prep time: 20 minutes
Cook time: 45 minutes
Servings: 9

Ingredients:

- 1 large egg, lightly beaten
- 2 cups of reduced-fat ricotta cheese
- 2 cups of shredded part-skim mozzarella cheese divided
- 4 oz crumbled feta cheese
- 1/4 cup of grated Parmesan cheese
- 1/4 cup of chopped fresh basil
- 2 garlic cloves, minced
- 1/4 teaspoon pepper
- 1 jar (24 oz) pasta sauce
- 9 no-cook lasagna noodles
- 3 cups of fresh baby spinach

Instructions:

1. Set the oven temperature to 350 degrees. Combine the following ingredients: egg, ricotta, feta, Parmesan, pepper, garlic, and 1/2 cup of mozzarella cheese.
2. Once oiled, spread 1/2 cup of spaghetti sauce into a 13x9-inch baking dish. Assemble the lasagna by layering three noodles, three quarters of a cup of ricotta mixture, one cup of spinach, and two thirds of a cup of sauce. Apply two more layers. Finish with a sprinkle of the leftover mozzarella.
3. Tend to the oven for thirty-five minutes while set covered. Turn the oven off and let the lasagna cook for another 10 to 15 minutes or until the cheese has melted. After 5 minutes, set aside to cool.

Pork Stir-Fried Noodles

Prep time: 5 minutes
Cook time: 15 minutes
Servings: 4

Ingredients:

- tablespoon of cider vinegar
- Two tablespoons of low-sodium soy sauce
- 1-tablespoon cornflour
- honey, one tablespoonful
- finely grated ginger, 1 teaspoon
- Strips of 400g of pork fillet
- 250 grams of hard-cooked egg noodles
- 1 tablespoon of coconut oil
- 1 sliced red pepper (without seeds)
- one hundred fifty grams of sliced mangetout
- 1 bunch of spring onions, peeled and cut into two halves: green and white
- Peel and slice one bunch of spring onions in half lengthwise; separate the white and green parts.
- 20 grams of roasted sesame seeds

Instructions:

1. Whisk the cornflour, vinegar, soy sauce, honey, and grated ginger together in a big basin. Mix in the pork slices until they are well coated. Put away to soak for a little while.
2. Toss the noodles with the boiling water in a bowl. After 10 minutes, remove from heat.
3. Warm up a big wok in a skillet over high heat before adding the vegetable oil. Once the smoke begins to rise, include the sliced pepper, mangetout, and white portions of the spring onions. Stir-fry for a minute, then toss in the pork strips that have been marinated; discard any excess marinade. After 3 to 4 minutes, stir-fry more.
4. Before adding to the pan, loosen the marinade by mixing 5 tablespoons of the noodle soaking water with the rest. Once the pork is halfway done, continue to stir-fry for

another two or three minutes. When the spring onions are still green, add them and turn off the heat.

5. Just before throwing in the meat and veggies, drain the noodles and throw them into the skillet. Toss with the toasted sesame seeds and chopped chilli before serving.

Italian-style Beef Meatballs

Prep time: 5 minutes
Cook time: 25 minutes
Servings: 16

Ingredients:

- A pound of lean ground beef, divided into four equal portions
- half a cup of marinara sauce.
- ¼ cup of Italian-seasoned breadcrumbs
- 2 cloves garlic, minced
- 1/4 cup of onion, grated
- 1 egg
- ¼ tsp dried oregano
- 3/4 tsp kosher salt
- ¼ tsp black pepper
- 2 tbsps fresh parsley, chopped
- Marinara sauce for serving

Instructions:

1. Adjust the oven temperature to 375 degrees Fahrenheit.
2. In a small food processor or cheese grater, mince the onion. The garlic should be minced. Remove the parsley leaves and stems.
3. Mix the meat, carrots, garlic, egg, breadcrumbs, oregano, salt, pepper, and parsley in a dish with the marinara sauce. Taste and season with pepper.
4. Blend the ingredients together using your hands.
5. Eighteen uniform servings should be made using a tiny scoop. Mold them into balls by rolling them with your palms.
6. An aerosol of olive oil should be lightly applied on a baking sheet.
7. Distribute the meatballs evenly on the baking sheet.
8. Place in the oven and cook for 20 to 25 minutes or until done.
9. Drizzle with more marinara sauce before serving.
10. Follow these steps to prepare a frying pan: heat it up over medium-high heat. While the meatballs are not yet cooked through, coat them with olive oil spray and sear them in a skillet over medium heat until they become golden brown. Use tongs to carefully turn the meatballs over. Toss them with the marinara sauce in a saucepan and simmer until they're done.

Pineapple Teriyaki Beef

Prep time: 10 minutes
Cook time: 10 minutes
Servings: 6

Ingredients:

- 1 ½ ibslib beef Top Sirloin Steak - cut into 1.5-inch pieces
- 2 cups of pineapple chunks
- 1 cup of prepared Teriyaki sauce
- sesame seeds - for garnish
- diced green onions - for garnish

Instructions:

1. In a medium-sized bowl, mix the steak with half of the teriyaki sauce and coat well. For 10 minutes, cover and refrigerate.
2. Use skewers to spear fruit and sirloin.
3. To get the doneness you prefer, which may range from medium rare (145°F) to medium (160°F) according to an instant-read thermometer, grill over medium heat for 3–4 minutes before turning and grilling for a further 3–4 minutes.
4. If you'd like, you may top it with sesame seeds and green onions and drizzle it with reserved Teriyaki sauce. Savour it!

Pork and Bean Casserole

Prep time: 10 minutes
Cook time: 30 minutes
Servings: 6

Ingredients:

- 1 can vegetarian baked beans 28 ozs
- Eight hot dogs, thinly cut into bite-sized portions
- Tomatoes, diced, 14.5 oz (drained)
- 1 cup of diced sweet yellow onion
- 1 cup of shredded Fiesta blend cheese, sometimes called Mexican blend cheese
- 1 package refrigerated jumbo biscuit dough 16 ozs/8 biscuits
- Alternatively, you may use heavy cream or butter and whisk in an egg for an egg wash.

Instructions:

1. Combine the beans, hot dogs, tomato, and onion in a 9" x 13" casserole dish.
2. Shredded cheese atop.
3. Take the dough out of the tube and flatten each biscuit with your fingers or a rolling pin. Form them so they fit in the pan and cover the dish. Making the biscuits thinner ensures that they will cook all the way through.
4. The whisked egg may be optionally used to coat the top of each cookie.
5. To get biscuits that are cooked through and have a golden brown top, place them on the center rack of an uncovered 350-degree oven and bake for about 30 minutes.

Beef and Potato Curry

Prep time: 15 minutes
Cook time: 1 hour 40 minutes
Servings: 4

Ingredients:

· 500g/17.5oz of stewing beef, raw
· 400g/14oz of baby potatoes, halved
· 1 onion, finely chopped
· 2 cloves of garlic, crushed
· 2 teaspoons of grated ginger
· 1 teaspoon of turmeric
· 1 tbsp of cumin seeds
· 1 tbsp of ground coriander
· 1 teaspoon of garam masala
· 1 green chilli, chopped

· 4 cardamom pods
· 4 cloves
· 4 Roma tomatoes, peeled and chopped
· 1 cup of/240ml of passata
• cup of beef broth (or 360 milliliters of water)
· amount of chopped spinach, around a handful
· An oil spray
· seasoned with salt & pepper

Instructions:

1. Coat a large saucepan with spray oil and place it over medium heat.
2. Fry the onion until it becomes tender.
3. Fry for a few more minutes after adding the turmeric, cumin seeds, ginger, and garlic.
4. Coat the beef well with the spices by adding the chopped tomatoes, coriander, cloves, chilli, cardamom pods, garam masala, and stirring.
5. Once again, bring to a boil. After that, reduce heat to low, cover, and simmer for fifteen minutes. Add the stock and passata and stir to combine. Halfway through, pause to see whether more materials are needed.
6. During the last half hour of cooking, toss in the potatoes.
7. After everything is cooked, mix in the spinach.
8. Use salt and black pepper to season as desired.
9. Add the sides of your choice and serve.

Honey Soy Glazed Beef Ribs

Prep time: 1 hour 5 minutes
Cook time: 40 minutes
Servings: 3

Ingredients:

• 5cm piece ginger, grated

• 6 garlic cloves, finely chopped

- 1/2 cup of (125ml) light soy sauce
- 1/2 cup of (175g) honey
- 1/2 cup of (125ml) Chinese rice wine (Shao Hsing - see notes)
- 1 tbsp sweet chilli sauce
- 1.4kg pork ribs cut into individual ribs
- Coriander sprigs to serve
- Lime wedges to serve

Instructions:

1. In a big zip-lock bag, combine the shredded ginger (5 cm), finely chopped garlic cloves (6 cloves), 1/2 cup of light soy sauce (125 ml), 1/2 cup of honey (175 g), 1/2 cup of Chinese rice wine (Shao Hsing; see notes) (125 ml), and 1 tablespoon of sweet chili sauce. Before sealing the bag, give the 1.4 kg of pork ribs a good shake to coat them evenly. Put in the fridge to marinate for at least an hour, or better yet, all night.
2. Bake at 180 degrees Celsius. While setting the ribs on a rack on a roasting pan with 1 cm of water, remove the marinade from the bag and put it aside. Carefully roast for 35 to 40 minutes or until golden caramel forms. After taking the pork off the rack, place it aside, loosely wrapped with foil, while you prepare the glaze.
3. Whisk together the marinade and any roasting pan juices in a small saucepan and set aside over medium-high heat to make the glaze. To make the mixture sticky, bring to a boil and then gently simmer for four to five minutes, stirring occasionally to prevent burning. Lightly coat the ribs with the glaze.
4. Hot ribs should be served with lime wedges and cilantro sprigs.

Pork and Cabbage Dumplings

Prep time: 30 minutes
Cook time: 10 minutes
Servings: 24

Ingredients:

- 5 oz cabbage napa or white (5oz is approx 1 ½ cups of shredded)
- 2 scallions spring onions
- ½ lb ground pork pork mince
- 1 tbsp soy sauce
- 1 teaspoon sesame oil
- 1 teaspoon Shaoxing wine or can use sherry
- ½ teaspoon ginger minced/finely grated
- 1 ½ tbsp cilantro/coriander, a small handful roughly chopped
- ¼ teaspoon salt
- 24 dumpling wrappers approx
- soy sauce with a little black vinegar or sriracha for dipping or your choice of dipping sauce.

Instructions:

1. Put the cabbage in a saucepan with some boiling water and blanch it for a few minutes to make it tender. Finely chop the cabbage. After draining, set aside for a few minutes to allow the cabbage to cool naturally.
2. While that's happening, thinly slice the scallions lengthwise and add them to the pork along with the rest of the ingredients (beyond the wrappers and sauce): soy sauce,

sesame oil, rice wine, ginger, cilantro, and salt. Thoroughly incorporate all of the ingredients; you may find that mixing by hand works best for this task.

3. Before adding the cabbage to the pork, squeeze it out as much moisture as you can using your hands or a towel. Roughly slice it. Thoroughly combine the ingredients.

4. Spoon some pork mixture over one side of a dumpling wrapper at a time, leaving a little space around the edge but generally filling it pretty completely. Make sure the edge of the wrapper is damp before folding it in half to connect it to the center, enclosing the filling. As you seal the dumpling edge from center to tip, squeeze or fold one side a few times with your thumbs and forefingers to create pleats along the edge. A video could be helpful in showing how to fold. Then, repeat the process on the other side. Fold the dumpling carefully so that it does not get trapped in too much air. Verify that the edge is securely sealed as well.

5. In a skillet or frying pan set over medium heat, warm up one or two teaspoons of oil for the classic dumpling recipe. Next, distribute the dumplings evenly around the pan. Cook for around two or three minutes to get a browned bottom. Boil enough water to cover the dumplings by three-quarters of the way up before placing a lid on top. Add about a quarter to a third cup of water to the pan. While the dumplings are boiling, the water will evaporate and become translucent. Brown the bases a little more after taking the lid off if you want them to be crispier.

6. To avoid sticking while steaming, line a bamboo steamer with paper or a cabbage leaf and arrange the dumplings closely together, leaving some space between each. Then, cook them until they are soft. Before placing over a pan or wok of boiling water, cover. The dumplings should be steam-cooked for three to four minutes or until they become transparent. As a side note, brown the underside of the item in a skillet or frying pan with 1 to 2 tablespoons of oil.

7. Serve with your preferred dipping sauce or soy sauce with a dash of sriracha or as a standalone condiment.

<u>Conclusion</u>

As I wrap up "The Galveston Diet Cookbook for Beginners," I want you to take a moment to think about all we've covered so far. Not only have we looked at recipes, but also a way of life—one that is balanced, healthy, and encourages wellbeing. When this book is closed, the reader has more than simply recipes; they have the means to begin a life-altering quest for healthier food and greater health.

A better living is the goal of this cookbook, not a random assortment of dishes. What matters most is embracing natural, unprocessed foods and taking pleasure in cooking tasty food that feeds the mind and spirit. We have stressed the significance of paying attention to our body when eating, being conscious of portion control, and making decisions that support our health objectives across these pages.

Beyond its culinary merits, "The Galveston Diet Cookbook for Beginners" exemplifies the transformative potential of camaraderie and mutual aid. Gathering around a table to eat, tell tales, and rejoice in life's little pleasures is what it's all about. Making bonds—with food, with one another, and with ourselves—is the point.

As the author, my wish is that this book will motivate readers to be more active in their own health care, to try different foods, and to appreciate the art of cooking. Above all else, I pray they keep in mind that being healthier isn't a race to perfection, but rather a marathon to progress. A lifetime of healthy habits may be yours with only a few simple, long-term adjustments.

Even though we're saying goodbye to "The Galveston Diet Cookbook for Beginners," we should take its wisdom with us as we go on in our lives and in the kitchen. Let us relish every second, every mouthful, and every chance to nurture ourselves and the people we care about. We have the ability to improve our health, one tasty meal at a time, so let's not lose sight of that.